FERTILITY SECRETS:

What Your Doctor Didn't Tell You About Baby-Making

Heal Your Body, Mind, and Spirit, Own Your Fertility, and Prepare for the Family of Your Dreams

By
Dr. Aumatma Shah

Published by Best Seller Publishing®, Pasadena, CA
Best Seller Publishing® is a registered trademark
Printed in the United States of America.
ISBN 978-1-946978-32-5

This publication is designed to provide accurate and authoritative information with regard to the subject matter covered. It is sold with the understanding that the publisher is not engaged in rendering legal, accounting, or other professional advice. If legal advice or other expert assistance is required, the services of a competent professional should be sought. The opinions expressed by the authors in this book are not endorsed by Best Seller Publishing® and are the sole responsibility of the author rendering the opinion.

Most Best Seller Publishing® titles are available at special quantity discounts for bulk purchases for sales promotions, premiums, fundraising, and educational use. Special versions or book excerpts can also be created to fit specific needs.

For more information, please write:
Best Seller Publishing®
1346 Walnut Street, #205
Pasadena, CA 91106
or call 1(626) 765 9750
Toll Free: 1(844) 850-3500
Visit us online at: www.BestSellerPublishing.org

I dedicate this book to my mother, for being my first example of the feminine, and to the love of my life who has supported me in birthing this book and helped me re-embrace and embody the feminine within myself.

I also dedicate it to my future child and the sons and daughters of the world, who are born to the strong, powerful women leading the way to re-embrace the feminine within.

Table of Contents

Introduction

Have you been trying to get pregnant for quite some time but not managed to conceive? Have you sought medical help that proved unfruitful? Do you feel like you are at your wit's end on your fertility journey? If so, you are not alone. In the U.S., one in eight couples between the ages of 18 and 35 has difficulty getting pregnant. That number increases after 35, as fertility is considered to decline considerably after 35. The fertility journey is often overshadowed by confusion, grief, frustration, and anxiety. What does it mean to be infertile? What can you do to get pregnant?

If you're like most of my clients, you have tried and tried, you've been to Dr. Google, frantically searching for the answer, the key to unlocking the mystery, and you're frustrated with your doctor, who only has a few very reserved answers for you. Usually, the first answer from your ob-gyn is to try Clomid. Next, it's on to cycle after cycle of intra-uterine insemination (IUI). And if that doesn't work, it's on to in-vitro fertilization (IVF). If your team is progressive, they might propose that you get acupuncture along with the cycles of IUI or IVF. But the truth is "infertility" is an umbrella label and doesn't tell you much about how you can treat it or support yourself in increasing your fertility.

I'm a naturopathic doctor and have been helping women with their health, vitality, and fertility for 10 years. For the last four, my practice has focused solely on fertility because I realize how much of a commitment it is to start a family, and I have seen the lack of options available to women and couples struggling with infertility. I have dedicated a lot of time to create a program that truly supports women *and* their partners to bring their health into an optimally fertile state. Following the program and improving their health and vitality, while addressing the root causes of their fertility struggles, help them to conceive easily and carry the child to term.

I'm passionate about this work because I have had my own journey and questions about fertility. At age 32, I was in a relationship with someone I potentially could have had children with, but I realized I didn't want to have children with him. And I knew fertility to some extent might decline with age. As we grow older, some changes in the body make it harder to conceive and carry to term, and we need to accept that. And the stats of age-related decline in fertility are conventionally rooted in the increasing risk of doing amniocentesis (at one time, the only diagnostic way to assess the fetus), which causes an increased risk of fetal death with increased maternal age. There is also evidence of declining values of anti-Müllerian hormone (AMH) with age. I was scared; how was I going to find a new partner and have babies before age 35 when conventional medicine proposes the decline of fertility?

Our Society's Approach to Baby-Making

I started doing some research and was disturbed by what I discovered. The media and doctors repeatedly warn women about their age-related fertility decline, yet corporations want women to wait till later to start families. A few years later, Facebook in Silicon Valley was one of the first companies to announce an unbeatable perk of working with them: Women were now going to have the option of freezing their eggs so they could work till later in life before deciding to settle down and procreate.

More and more women do choose to wait till later in life to start families. Some delay it because of their careers; some do it because they have not found the perfect partner for it yet, and some do it because their partners are not ready to commit till later in life. Just to offer you some perspective, my grandmother was married at the age of 14 and had seven children between 14 and 30. Compare that to my mother, who had two children between 27 and 30. Most of the women I work with are over 35.

In the last three generations, there have been drastic changes, and these have brought about challenges. We have had to step up and create new responses to these challenges, and we have! The progress in reproductive technologies has given women options when it comes to starting a family.

Egg freezing is an innovative and revolutionary technology, but the statistics surrounding it need to be brought to light. Of all the eggs that are frozen every year that are thawed to use for reproduction, there is a 77% failure rate in 30-year-old women and a 91% failure rate in 40-year-old women. The American Society of Reproductive Medicine (ASRM) cautions against the use of egg freezing for the purpose of delaying childbearing. I consider egg freezing to be a young, yet potentially promising technology for those who have the resources. It may be a reasonable backup plan, but it should not be mistaken for a failsafe.

Another option that is available today is reproduction through in-vitro fertilization (IVF); however, this approach is also extremely masculine in the way it tries to control and overpower the natural rhythm and flow of hormones in the body. Though IVF is a great tool and could be a necessity for some, many women think of it as a way to conceive whenever they want to. This may not sound too bad, and it could be a route that some women choose. But problems arise when a woman expects that IVF will help her magically get pregnant whenever she wants to and it doesn't work. Many women have been fooled to believe that with IVF, they would get pregnant the very first month they decided they were ready to start a family. The fact is that only 24% of IVF cycles result in successful conception, and not all of those result in live births. The average success rate of a fertility treatment at a reproductive clinic is roughly 24% for any given *ideal* cycle. Stated differently, out of the 1.5 million IVF procedures that are performed per year, 1.2 million result in failure.[1]

Though there is an average published rate of decline in fertility with age, the rates of conception with assisted reproductive technologies (ART) are not drastically better than the rates of natural conception.

Age	Fertility Rates	Fertility Rates with Medical Intervention (based on average published rates by CDC)
<30	28.5%	36.6%
31-35	21.5%	36.6%
35-37	16.3%	30%
38-40	9.1%	20%
41-43	4.1%	10.7%
40-45	2%	3.5%

[1]   Tsigdinos, P. M. (2014, October 24). The Sobering Facts About Egg Freezing That Nobody's Talking About. Retrieved July 24, 2017, from https://www.wired.com/2014/10/egg-freezing-risks/

As you can see from this chart, the rates with ART methods, such as IVF, are sometimes only 2–6% higher than the rates of natural conception within given age groups.

Don't get me wrong; I think ART is brilliant and an incredible technology. I do believe, however, that it's most helpful for a small percentage of people with particular issues. For example, it is a necessity for women with physical issues such as blocked fallopian tubes, hydrosalpinx, and more. ART is not the magical answer for everyone, though.

It nagged me that in the scientific world, there was an overwhelming belief that age determined fertility success, and that the women I talked to held an almost opposing belief that with IVF or frozen eggs, they could live how they wanted until they were ready to have children.

Where Was the Voice of Women?

The big problem with all of what I was discovering was that all of the perks and research were coming from a male perspective. Where was the voice of women? Where was the Goddess who represented true human potential? I saw very little belief in the empowered woman— belief that we perhaps could learn how to care for and be in tune with our bodies and our innate wisdom so that we could wait (within reason) to procreate at the time of our choice. I wanted us to claim back our power.

It was then that I rediscovered Christiane Northrup's book *Women's Bodies, Women's Wisdom*, which inspired me to think about age-related infertility in a different way. Dr. Northrup suggested that there were women in other, more remote parts of the world who could healthily conceive children at 60 years of age. So what were we in the Western society doing wrong? I went on a rampant search for "the answer," and I came to the conclusion that though our fertility is influenced by age, it is likely more impacted by stress, lifestyle, and underlying factors causing the reproductive system to shut down. Though I am in no way advocating to wait until age 45 to start trying, I believe that actively taking care of ourselves and our bodies, keeping our hormones in balance, and optimizing our lifestyle for fertility will help us preserve our fertility.

With my clients, we don't focus exclusively on conception. When the body is in balance, getting pregnant is easy. "Infertility" is just a label for a condition that can have many root causes. As a naturopathic doctor, I integrate the best of east and west. The truth is Western medicine is quite brilliant! It has many tools and ways of understanding the physiology and chemistry of the body, which, when used with curiosity, can give us some great information. In my clinic, we consider the treatment of a client to be successful if it clears the client's body of the blocks to pregnancy, rebalances the body and hormones, and heals the mind–body state so that conception can happen. My clients have achieved their targeted health goals 85% of the time, whether that be pregnancy or optimizing their health to a standard they set at treatment onset. The reason that this more holistic approach works so well is that we optimize the state of the body. It goes back to addressing the underlying causes in a holistic way—from a mind, body, and spirit perspective.

One Desire, Various Obstacles

One woman who came to me at age 34 had been told by her doctor to keep trying because everything looked normal. She had been trying for more than a year, though, and she hadn't conceived. She had been to acupuncture for over six months, her periods were regular, and there was no obvious reason that she was not getting pregnant. Western medicine said she was fine; Eastern medicine was addressing her "spleen qi deficiency" (a diagnosis in Chinese medicine that refers to a decreased flow of energy to and from the spleen organ and additionally implies a depleted energy of the entire digestive system), but she was not feeling any different, so she proceeded to look for other support. First, my patient went to the nutritionist who put her on a gluten-free diet. Then she went to the energy healer who she decided to work with regularly. Lastly, she checked in with a psychic to see if she would get pregnant soon. No one thus far understood what was happening. Did she have nutritional deficiencies? Were her hormones out of balance? Had the stress she has experienced in her life damaged her ovaries (reversibly)?

Another patient who came to me was a 38-year-old woman with high FSH (follicle stimulating hormone), low AMH (anti-Müllerian hormone), and low progesterone. She had been trying to conceive for three years. She had tried several rounds of IVF, done acupuncture, and taken the herbs and followed the diets. Nothing was working. Her reproductive endocrinologist could just suggest another round of IVF—maybe the next one would be more successful. She was frustrated and didn't know what to do. When she came to me, she was very upset about all the money she had spent and, even more importantly, the time she had spent. She and her husband had started having challenges both in the bedroom and outside of it. She felt worn out, and she was tired of having to time sex rather than letting it be spontaneously fun as it used to be. She was also tired of having to work on herself. On a deeper level, she felt like her body had failed her and something was wrong with her.

A third patient who sought my help was a 35-year-old woman who had had two miscarriages around Week 6 or 7. She felt a lot of grief from losing the first two pregnancies and blamed herself because she couldn't figure out why this would happen. Although her husband wanted to be supportive, she felt all alone and scared. Her doctor didn't have any suggestions for her—only told her that her next pregnancy might be different.

All three of these women were struggling with having the one thing they wanted more than anything else—a baby. This is a unique kind of want; it's a deep desire for procreation, for manifestation, for something deep within them that cannot be equaled to anything else. It's a calling to be a mother. These women came to me with very different underlying problems, but with my holistic approach of finding the root cause, detoxifying the body, rebalancing hormones and underlying physiology, and working on the mind–body–emotional connections, all three of these women were able to conceive successfully and have healthy babies.

For the first patient, it was hormonal imbalances that caused infertility. The doctors she went to never tested her; they assumed that things were fine. In reality, she had high AMH levels, slightly elevated testosterone, and high LH (luteinizing hormone), which indicated that she likely had polycystic ovary syndrome or PCOS for short. We will talk more about PCOS later. Since they didn't test her, she went for months not understanding why she wasn't conceiving. Had she known that she had PCOS, which caused her body not to ovulate, she could have taken some action steps to help bring her body into some hormonal balance. Once we established that she did have PCOS, we utilized herbal medicines that helped bring her hormones in balance, and that made her cycles more regular. We also used Myo-Inositol, which has been researched to support healthy ovulation, even better than metformin in some studies! A mere six months later, she conceived naturally and went on to have a healthy baby.

The second patient came into my office with a binder full of lab tests. She had been to several specialists and had done many tests. I found her FSH at 18 to be a little high, but not horrible. And her AMH was low at 0.35, but I had seen those numbers change in prior patients, so I was not too concerned about them. I was more concerned about her mind–body state and her frustration, anger, and fear.

In her specialized program, we focused primarily on healing and rebuilding. We increased her nutritional levels based on functional testing and addressed the underlying inflammation that was present in her body. We also rebalanced her body from years of stress with mind–body techniques and herbs. In addition, we did a hands¬-on therapy called Mercier Therapy. Mercier Therapy is a deep manipulation (based on osteopathy) of the reproductive organs, as well as loosening of the muscles in the buttocks, which help to unwind the ligament attachments of the ovaries. Restoring fluidity in the reproductive organs supports the ovaries to have better blood flow and positioning. Studies have shown that 80% of women between the ages of 35 and 45 who undergo Mercier Therapy treatment are successful in conceiving naturally or through IVF within one year of treatment. This therapy helped physically shift the location of this patient's uterus and ovaries and increase the blood flow and circulation to the area, which supported optimal baby-making. Last but not least, we zoned in on nutrients that would help increase the quality of her eggs, which supported a natural increase in her progesterone levels.

Four months later, her lab values were normal. Taking her age into account, they could even be considered great! After that, she tried to conceive naturally for three cycles but didn't succeed. At that point, she decided it was time for her to try a more integrative approach, so she went to a local IVF clinic for her fourth round. Even though she had tried several rounds of IVF unsuccessfully before, this time was different. She was in a more balanced state, many more eggs were retrieved, and as she was more relaxed, she was better situated to receive the embryos. We continued the mind–body sessions because she said they kept her more calm and positive. Sure enough, one of the embryos implanted, and voila! She was pregnant. Not only that; she had a healthy baby, and the work we did through her pregnancy helped her have an easeful birth and adapt quickly and easily post-partum.

The third patient's predicament was a bit different. She had no problem getting pregnant but was unable to carry to term. When she reached out to me, she wasn't sure if I could help her, since I was a fertility specialist, not a miscarriage specialist. Repeated pregnancy loss is, however, as much of a fertility issue as is the inability to conceive, because the root cause is often similar. I have had many repeat pregnancy loss patients, and there can be different underlying reasons for each one's issue. This patient likely had a progesterone deficiency that couldn't be addressed by taking extra progesterone (she had already tried that in her second pregnancy).

I am not a proponent of blind progesterone usage, especially in younger women, since it is frequently found that low progesterone levels are a result of poor egg quality,[2] so our approach was a little different. First and foremost, she and her husband were to take a break from baby-making. They needed *not* to get pregnant while we were addressing some of the root cause imbalances. Then we started increasing her egg quality, improving the positioning of her uterus and ovaries through Mercier Therapy, and flooding her body with nutrients. We also found that she had a heterozygous genetic defect that caused mal-absorption and mal-utilization of folic acid. With a deeper look, we found many defects in her genetic pathways that needed to be addressed. Also, her husband worked in a high-stress environment and needed some holistic support to increase the nutrient levels in his body and raise his vitality.

They wanted to fast-track their program, so they completed the fertility success program in three months. Two weeks after finishing the program, they got pregnant. She was scared when she got the positive pregnancy test because she hadn't planned to get pregnant

---

[2] Hannam, T. (2014, December 26). "How does my menstrual cycle reflect the quality of my eggs?" [Web log post]. Retrieved July 24, 2017, from http://fertility.ca/eggs/menstrual-cycle-reflect-quality-eggs/

that quickly. We continued with mind–body support through the first trimester of her pregnancy and a couple of check-in and rebalancing appointments in the second and third trimester. She was able to carry to term and gave birth to a healthy baby girl.

A Template for Learning

Each of these patients and couples are unique. Their stories are unique, and so is yours. One of the couples I mentioned above might resonate with you. There is, however, no magic formula or pill that I can suggest for everyone across the board. Everyone needs different things, and no one remedy or special fertility diet can fit all. Also, there is no super food that will magically help you get pregnant. There are many foods that have gone through their five minutes of fame, such as maca, cacao, and acai, but none of them will last because even though each one can help women with particular imbalances, no one herb or supplement is going to be the magic fix. Some of these can actually throw you more off-balance, so I suggest seeking expert guidance rather than going down the track of self-prescribing or using Dr. Google to treat you.

There is, nevertheless, a template for learning about the body and understanding it that can help with conception and healthy birth. More than magic pills and bullets, this book is about a path, a journey, and a perspective you can carry with you. I will show you some pieces you might be missing for understanding the underlying causes of your challenge in conceiving. I will also show you how you can empower yourself with the knowledge to integrate your body, mind, and spirit. In addition, I will teach you about the energies that get in the way of conception and the physiology that brings discord to your baby-making.

My mission with this book, as well as my practice, is to empower you to choose to have children when you want to. I want to show you how you can prepare and optimize your body and bring it into balance, whether you are actively trying to conceive or you want to preserve your fertility for later. I believe that every woman should have this information about her body and hormones and be empowered to take charge of it in a way that is supportive of health and fertility for the long run. That way, you can have children when you're ready to and it's an easy process when you make the decision to do so. That doesn't mean I think women are invincible or are unaffected by age. It just means that to me, having a child is a conscious choice, and sometimes you don't know when you will make that choice. But when you get there, you should have a place to turn to and get guidance.

In addition, with this book, I want to help you reclaim the feminine on the journey of fertility that has been overtaken by masculine approaches to health and healing. The approach and path I share in this book are all about embracing our flow and the feminine to live healthier, more fulfilling lives—and making choices that are in alignment with our bodies, which can be helpful in conceiving now or preserving your fertility till later.

If you have the chance to freeze your eggs, do it. But preserve the eggs inside your body to the best of your ability as well. And if you already are at the point of trying IVF or having failed several cycles of IVF, don't worry. It's not your fault that you have bought into the belief that IVF will be your saving grace—it's what you have been told by the media and the doctors you trust. That belief is what has driven so many women to try cycle after cycle of IVF, without stopping to wonder, "How is doing the same thing again and again going to lead to a different outcome?" In fact, Albert Einstein once said the definition of insanity is "doing the same thing again and again and expecting a different outcome."

There are undoubtedly plenty of stories of women who have successfully had babies via IVF. But it is not the perfect answer for everyone. So how do you know when you should try something different? How do you know which approach might work best for you? Before you spend $20,000 to $25,000 *per cycle* of IVF, I highly recommend figuring out if you actually need it or if you're doing it out of fear. You know the adage, "If all you have is a hammer, everything looks like a nail." If your doctor only has a hammer as a mode of treatment, you will be that nail. I suggest finding a doctor who has a hammer, a screwdriver, and a wrench in his or her toolkit.

My intention throughout this book is to unearth truths that are not shared in the mainstream paradigms so that you can best understand your body and the fluctuations of hormones. You will be able to help uncover the root cause of your infertility so you can help heal at the root, instead of trying to control and overpower.

I want to help bring you in sync with your power so that you can choose the best route to baby-making for you. The question I encourage women to ask themselves is this: Does the approach of doing whatever you want, treating your body however you want, pumping it full of hormones to prevent pregnancy and then pumping it full of hormones when you want to have a baby, support your highest manifestation of the feminine? Does this get you closer to understanding and being in rhythm with your body? Or does it have you shut down your body's natural rhythms and bring you closer to a more masculine state?

I believe that either way you choose is fine, but I also believe that we as a culture would benefit from a reconnection with our feminine. As I look around the world, I feel like we are in dire need of more feminine energy. And, on a personal level, I have seen women transform their lives by reconnecting with the feminine.

As you read on and dive deeper into your fertility, I encourage you to take what resonates with you and leave what doesn't.

If you want to move from feeling frustrated, angry, and lost as to where to turn next to having an integrated, wholesome knowledge of your body¬–mind and feeling empowered to make choices based on your values rather than fear, this is your book! My hope is that every chapter in this book leaves you feeling a little more inspired and with a few more tools. In addition, I have included lots of bonuses you can to download. These are practical tools you can start applying to optimize your body and increase your fertility right away. May you get exactly what you need from this book and may you conceive naturally or find yourself releasing what stands in the way of you conceiving and having the family you have always dreamed of.

Guide through the Book

There are a few things I should tell you as you dive in. First and foremost, there was a lot of information that I feel is important for your fertility that I wanted you to have, but as it didn't allow the book to flow the way I wanted it to, I have put it into a *Fertility Secrets Bonus Kit* with several free downloads that I mention throughout the book. You can have them all at once by going to this link: http://www.draumatma.com /fertility-secrets-bonuses/, opting in, and downloading it.

Second, this book is organized by mind–body connections first. These are based on the themes I have noticed and realizations I have had by being in practice for over 10 years. This is what is most exciting for me to share with you. The magical stories that I have experienced through the eyes of my patients are priceless. I hope you will find hope and joy in these stories, as well as reflections of things you experience in your own life. The second half of the book is all the scientific, research-based content that I am sure will give you the answers you have been looking for. In the last month alone, I have had over 15 women say that a 30-minute conversation with me resulted in more answers than they had been able to find by talking to multiple experts in the fertility field. I have attempted to transmit all of my knowledge into this book, but if you feel like you need to talk to someone, I offer 30-minute video consults on my website. For now, they are completely free, but I imagine that if my schedule gets to over-booked, I might have to start charging a nominal fee for them. You can schedule a consult here: http://www.draumatma.com/schedule-an-appt/. Please remember to choose Option 2, Video Consult for Fertility/ Hormonal Challenges if you want to have the consult with me. Otherwise, I have another doctor working with me who can also help.

Last but not least, connect with me! I want to hear what insights you're having, breakthroughs you're creating in your life, and babies you're manifesting as you move through this book. I have created a closed group on Facebook called Fertility Secrets. Join me there so we can connect in real time!

CHAPTER 1

Start with the Why

One would think that the fertility journey would support intimacy, but it can do quite the opposite. Beginning their fertility journey, many couples are bright-eyed, bushy-tailed, starters. As they progress, though, it wears on them and their relationship. Women typically feel frustrated and alone in the relationship while men often feel that they're being used for their sperm. It puts a lot of pressure on the couples and often ends up causing them to lose intimacy when all they want is to have a family and feel supported in the process. Couples that have tried to get pregnant for a while often fear that their relationship might fall apart if conception doesn't happen, and sometimes that fear might turn out to be true.

I once worked with a couple where the wife deeply wanted a child, but the husband was quite uninterested. When they came to me, she was excited to start the program. He, on the other hand, didn't care whether or not they had a child; he just thought his wife would leave him if they didn't, and since they were in their 40s, it was now or never. Since he didn't care, he didn't want to make time for the program, and he even skipped appointments. Eventually, it became apparent that they were fighting and blaming each other. They never got on the same page, and they ended up discontinuing the program because they lost their way in the midst of their relationship.

Get the Right Mindset

Before you embark on the fertility journey, you must prepare yourself so that if this journey becomes challenging, it brings you closer to your spouse rather than disconnected from each other and frustrated. An important part of the preparation is getting the right mindset. This is easier for some couples to achieve than others.

I recommend starting with the *why*. Simon Sinek has a TED Talk where he does an excellent job illustrating the importance of determining your *why* called "How Great Leaders Inspire." In this discussion, he uses Apple as an example. Apple's *why* is to be the most cutting edge by challenging the status quo. As a result of starting with that *why*, buyers line up outside their stores to buy their products days before the products are released. While Sinek speaks from a business perspective, his principle is applicable to life in general. If you establish a solid understanding of your *why*, you will come up with a process that will help you achieve your goal and stay committed to that path. Establishing your *why* will help you and your partner get on the same page. If you are already on the same page, you can talk about what else you want to incorporate into the process. This is just the tip of the iceberg, and you can dig deeper as you explore this. In the midst of any discomfort or relationship struggle that may arise along the way, you can come back to the *why*. You can also come back to it if frustration and lack of hope cause you to want to quit trying and forget all about babies. So *why* do you want to have a baby?

Ground Yourself and Create a Strong Intention

After you have identified your *why*, you want to create a strong intention—a statement of what you would like the process to be like. Your *why* is essentially your vision statement. It's what your life would be like if you had it all your way, and that is what you want to manifest. To manifest it—to create that life you want to live—you need to create that strong intention.

Before you create this intention, spend a few minutes grounding yourself. If you don't believe in meditation, you can skip this step. One way of grounding yourself is by putting your hand over your abdomen and inhaling slowly and deeply a few times. You can also sit on a chair or the floor and imagine a cord going from the bottom of your buttocks to the center of the earth. This cord can be made of anything—light, crystals, or even leather; it's your choice. I often use the trunk of a tree because that feels very earthy to me. Imagine this cord coming out of your seat bottom and going down into the center of the earth. It can go as deep as you can imagine it. Then widen this cord to at least the width of your body. Double the width of your body is even better. Imagining this massive trunk or tremendous force of energy will help you feel solid and grounded in your body. You can bring this cord from your bottom up to your head to ground the mind as well. People often complain that they can't meditate because their minds are constantly racing. If you bring this cord all the way up to your head, it will quiet your mind and bring you in the right space to do the rest of the exercise.

Once you are grounded, you can create the intention. Rather than making the intention all about your goal of having a baby, make it about your journey and who you want to become in the process. Get into the feelings of it. An example might be, "I intend to be guided to learning more about myself and my partner in the process of having a healthy child." If you want, you can articulate it in the form of a prayer: "I pray that I get clarity to remove any blocks to having a baby." Most importantly, put it in your own words and tap into your deepest intentions for being on the fertility path.

Make a Vision Board

The next step is to create a vision board. Make one for yourself and invite your partner to do the same. You could also create a vision board together. There are many ways to create a vision board. I recommend collecting random magazines (not just baby-related ones) and cutting out pictures and words that stand out to you. If you have a strong intention and are grounded in yourself when you do it, you will find the things that stand out to you quite easily. Include all aspects of your life—your body, mind, and spirit. What does your ideal life look like? What will feed your body? What will feed your mind? What will feed your spirit? What do you wish to create in the process of having a baby? What else do you want to create in your life?

Here is an example of a vision board from one of my clients:

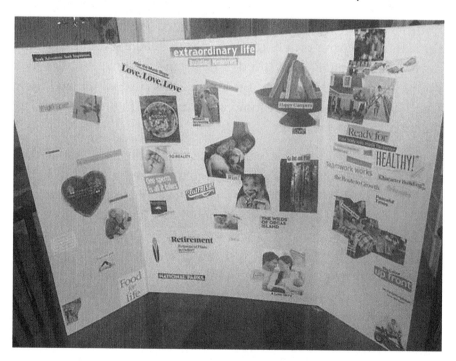

I have advised many couples to create vision boards, and many have said it was a bonding experience for them. Making boards separately and then seeing what the other has created has helped them get on the same page or stay on the same page if they already agreed on what they wanted.

Recently a set of my clients, a woman who was 40 and her husband who was 47, did this exercise. Once they had finished, the wife came to me and told me the exercise made her feel invigorated in the relationship because they had so many of the same things on their vision boards. She showed me a picture, and I could see how beautifully similar their boards were even though they had made them separately.

This practice can be helpful if you and your partner are on different pages regarding having a child or have different commitment levels of creating a family. Most couples on the fertility journey are united in their dedication to family-creation, but sometimes things can shift for one and not the other. So it's important to check in along the way and make sure there is a safe space where both of you can express your desires. If you discover that you are not in the same place, or you have mixed feelings about having a baby, it is important you find someone you can talk to who can support you in gaining clarity.

A few couples that started the fertility program with me hadn't checked in with each other first. When they had the time, space, and safety to do that, they were deeply relieved to discover that the other person felt like they did—no longer wanting to have a child. One couple had been trying to conceive for 10 years! Imagine their relief when they both discovered that their partner was ready to let go of having a child and create purpose around something else together! They were immensely grateful for the process and healing they received that allowed them to come to this conclusion. They were also very grateful to get their lives back rather than having put them on hold for some future moment that was going to be happier and better than the current one.

In either case, with the proper preparation, the process of having a child is an opportunity for you to connect with your partner and deepen the relationship.

CHAPTER 2

Letting Go of the "Why Me?"

The alarm buzzes—it's 6:59 a.m. "Time to take your temperature," says a reminder that pops up on her phone. It's Month 7 of thermometers, timed sex, and peeing on LH sticks to see if she's ovulating. As she lies there, thermometer in her mouth, she wonders, when will this end? Why can't I get pregnant? All my friends have had babies already—some even two by now. But here I am. What did I do wrong? Did I drink too much when I was in college? Maybe I'm too stressed out. But something is certainly wrong with me. Why me?

Why me? Why am I not pregnant yet? What did I do wrong? Should I have done something differently? Many women battle with these questions every day of their adult lives. All they want is to be able to have a baby and start a family without struggling, but they are unable to. One in eight women between the ages of 18 and 34 experiences infertility. Notice I said 18 and 34. This is a shocking statistic because most of the women I work with are over the age of 30. This demographic of women has an even higher rate of infertility. Women under age 35 need to have tried to conceive for at least one year unsuccessfully to be diagnosed as infertile. Women over 35 need to have tried unsuccessfully for at least six months. The question of "why me" often comes up when a couple has decided that they want to have a baby and have tried without success for some months. A majority of women will begin wondering if something is wrong with their bodies or start feeling like they are victims of their circumstances within the first three to six months of trying. Imagine that experience multiplied over three, four, or five years. Obviously, it is difficult.

The Intricate Process of Conception

Many women think they will get pregnant as soon as they decide they are ready to have a child; however, it doesn't work that way. In any given cycle in a woman's life, she has roughly a 25% chance of conceiving. That is a fairly low probability. It contradicts what many women are taught when they are young—that they *will* get pregnant if they have unprotected sex. They adopt this misconception and carry it with them throughout their lives, failing to understand that their bodies need to go through an intricate process to conceive.

Conception depends on a fine-tuned balance of thyroid hormones, adrenal hormones, follicle stimulating hormone, luteinizing hormone, estrogen, and progesterone; the process of egg and sperm production; and the chemokines necessary to combine the egg and sperm. It is a true miracle when conception happens!

First, let's consider egg and sperm development. At birth, women have 1 million eggs. By puberty, only 250,000 remain. Sperm take 75 to 90 days to be produced properly. So everything leading up to 90 days prior to conception significantly affects the sperm.

If the egg matures properly, it will be released from the ovary. Motivated by estrogen signals, it will go into the fallopian tube and float down into the middle where it will hope to meet the sperm.

Granted that the sperm are produced properly, many of them will enter from the vagina and go up the cervix into the fallopian tube. The harsh, acidic environment of the vagina will kill the majority of the sperm before they get to the cervix. In the cervix, the sperm will swim upstream and against the cilia that push against them. Out of the thousands that were released, only 30 or so sperm will make it into the fallopian tubes, and hopefully, they make it into the correct fallopian tube (the side on which the ovary released the egg this month). The egg only has a 36-hour window to be fertilized, so the sperm have to be present and ready to meet the egg.

As soon as the sperm get in the vicinity of the egg, they will try to penetrate the protective coating around the egg. They have to be strong enough to burrow through this protective layer. If a sperm makes it through this layer, it has succeeded. Then the egg and sperm will unite and begin their journey together as an embryo.

The newly formed embryo will travel down the fallopian tube into the uterus and implant there. At implantation, the right hormones have to exist for the embryo to "take" or physically merge and become embedded into the uterus, where it will grow for nine months.

The fact that all the pieces have to align perfectly even for the sperm and egg to meet, let alone implant and grow, makes the entire journey a miracle. For me, it's a journey of pure awe and wonder, and I'm amazed by the miracle of life. So please realize and understand that getting pregnant is a process. Just because it may take some time, it doesn't mean something is wrong with you.

A Spiritual Dimension

I once spoke at a conference of about 2,000 women. After I had finished the talk, one of the women came up to me and said, "Why am I struggling with this when so many women get pregnant at the drop of a hat? They don't do yoga, they eat crappy food, and they aren't doing anything for their health. Maybe they're even drinking alcohol every day or smoking cigarettes, and they still get pregnant. Here I am. I do yoga every day. I eat super healthy. I've been getting acupuncture for five years. But I'm still not pregnant. Why me?"

Many of the women I work with have similar stories. They are already living extremely healthy lives. They eat only organic food. They go to yoga every week. So what is it about these women, and why are so many women struggling with having children when women in other parts of the world don't live nearly as healthily but still manage to conceive?

After much contemplation, I came to the conclusion that there must be a deeper and more spiritual reason why they have not yet gotten pregnant. Though their lifestyle supports the health of their physical bodies, it could be that the spirits that want to come through them desire a deeper level of health by integrating the mind and body. More about this perspective can be found in the book *Spirit Babies* by Walter Makichen. The word *spirit* can be scary or triggering for some, so let me explain further what I mean. My belief, which is shared by the many people I work with, is that babies are spirits to start with. They exist in the ethereal realms before they choose the parents they will be born through. They may have picked a set of parents but want those parents to have a certain level of mental, physical, and spiritual well-being before they are born into the planet. Perhaps they have purposes that require their parents to be in a certain state of health. The spirit or the child-to-be might have a desire to help make the world a healthier and happier place, and to do that, it will need parents who are willing to support it. Then the baby spirit is simply preparing the parents to provide what it needs for a successful journey through childhood so that it can fulfill its purpose as an adult.

Or perhaps it is an opportunity for learning, self-discovery, and growth. A dear friend who had struggled with conceiving at the tender age of 29, said to me recently, "I learned so much about my body in the process of trying to conceive and carry a child to term that I am actually grateful. I wish that when I was 15 years old, I had been taught more about my body, hormones, and the process of conception instead of the teaching that it would be so easy to have a baby that even kissing could get you pregnant."

Another client of mine, who has been on the fertility journey for five years, has had major shifts in her energy through this journey, and now she is in a place of relaxation and being able to receive. She has moved from thinking, "Why me?" to "This is just what I needed." The path has inspired her to do something she never would have otherwise—she has started training to be a health coach, and one day she hopes to serve women like her who are going through what she went through on her fertility journey. She even said to me that if she had not had to deal with these challenges, she would not have been able to get to where she is now, and that the baby spirit that wants to come through her needed her to be in the mental-emotional-energetic space she is in now.

If the spiritual perspective doesn't resonate with you, that is okay. You don't have to adopt it. It might, however, give you an opportunity step away from the "why me" victim mentality and belief that you are being punished. Instead of thinking "why me," try shifting your perspective to "why not me" and acknowledge that there may be a gift in the midst of your struggle. Perhaps it produces in you a more balanced state of mind and body that can fully support the amazing spirit that wants to come through you! Or perhaps your perspective is that there is no big reason, that this is just your mountain to climb. That's a great perspective too.

If you often find yourself with the "why me" and "something must be wrong with me" perspective, though, it may be time to make a shift! As long as your point of view doesn't hold you back, it's great. Just consider it carefully and be honest with yourself.

I once had a client who sought my help at age 40. For months, I treated physiological issues she had such as hormone imbalances, food sensitivities, and more. However, it seemed like something remained out of balance. She always rushed to get to her next work meeting or phone call, or just rushed our appointments in general.

When I noticed her tendency to check her watch, I tried to ask her about her lifestyle and stress, but it wasn't until I saw the inside of her house that I understood. Her entire house was white with no hint of color anywhere—not on the cushions, not on the chairs, not on the table. Everything was white. She had exhibited some traits of a type-A personality before I visited her home, but after I had seen the inside of her house, it was clear to me that she was not ready for a child. I said to her, "How do you expect a child to live in this all-white environment? A child isn't going to think about keeping your couch clean or not getting your sheets dirty."

She thought about it for a minute. Then she responded, "Ha. I guess I've always been this way."

We dug a little deeper and discovered a pattern; throughout her life, she had wanted control in every aspect of her life. That included her partner who she was trying to have a baby with. She had been controlling him for the entirety of their relationship, and she said that he wasn't fully masculine and that she had to tell him what to do all the time. I saw that she needed to let go of her desire to be in control. If she could do that, she would very likely be able to shift the dynamic in her relationship and allow space for the baby spirit that wanted to be born by her.

Sure enough, two short weeks after she let go of the need to control everything, she became pregnant. Mind you, she had already been through three rounds of IVF before she started working with me. She had also been doing acupuncture for five years and ate extremely healthily. When she realized that she'd had this pattern her entire life, she didn't know she could shift it if she chose to. When I let her know that she had the power to make the change, she seized that power and did it. The shift from needing to control everything to being open to what the baby spirit wanted for their life together was an important step in solving her problem.

Embrace a New Mindset

If you ask yourself "why me," I would like you to think carefully about whether or not this question serves you. If it doesn't, I invite you to consider a few other questions in its place.

When you think "why me," you are in victim mode. Before you replace this question and way of thinking, take a moment to embrace it and allow it to be. There is nothing wrong with feeling however you feel at any given moment. Don't ignore it or push it away. The key is simply not to become stuck in that mode.

Once you have sat with it, and you feel like the charge of it has disappeared, you can shift to different questions such as "Why not me?" "What is this journey teaching me?" "What can I gain from the challenges I'm facing?" "Who do I have the opportunity to become?" "How am I bigger than this problem or challenge?" You may want to write down the thoughts that occur when you consider these questions. All of them are designed to help you dig a little bit deeper into the challenges you're facing and help you move away from "why me," which blocks the connection between your mind and body and deprives you of the power to choose and change. When you make this shift, you invite the process of integrating your mind and body.

The fertility journey can be beneficial in many ways, as it has been for my clients who were in search of happiness. Having a child is one way to find happiness, but my goal is always to help my clients feel happy even before they get pregnant. It's about living in the emotional state of already having achieved whatever your goal is. Also, my clients desire to hit the "unpause" button on life. They think, "After I have the positive pregnancy test, I'll feel happy. I'll feel free. I'll travel. I'll do all of the things I want to do." One of the biggest lessons infertility teaches women is to be more relaxed, let go more often, and re-embrace the feminine, which many us have been taught to shut down and throw into a corner.

CHAPTER 3

The Masculine–Feminine Spectrum

This chapter is about how we easily shift our roles and the way we are in a relationship, which is a topic I'm extremely passionate about because it's where my journey started. For most of my life, I was a tomboy, playing sports and hanging out with the "guys." I had many male friends but didn't get along with many women. Looking back, I believe I had shut down my feminine side because I was sexually abused at a young age. That also led me to yearn for spiritual realization, purpose, and the meaning of life at an early age. I did not, however, live in my body very often. My spirit usually floated about 20 feet outside of my body, and I was not very grounded. Without being grounded (which is the first chakra), it is impossible to be in the feminine (which is mostly second chakra energy).

You may be wondering, what are chakras? According to Vedic traditions from India, chakras are centers of energy. The Vedic philosophy says we have seven major energy centers and many more minor energy centers—all of which rule and govern different aspects of our mind–body–spirit connection.

The first, or root, chakra is the energy center that helps us feel grounded and rooted in this world. It can also be connected to survival. Common symptoms of a shut down first chakra are manifested as feelings of scarcity, problems with money, abundance, insecurities, and indecisiveness.

The second, or sacral, chakra is the energy center connected with sexual health and creativity. A block of creativity in the younger years can often lead to problems in the reproductive organs later in life.

The third, or solar plexus, chakra is the energy center connected with purpose and personal power. An imbalance in this chakra may result in a sense of lack of purpose or direction in life. This feeling may cause us to overcompensate by going out of our way to prove ourselves and find that source of power through approval from others. An imbalance in this chakra can also manifest itself in digestive issues.

The fourth, or heart, chakra is the energy center for love—both self-love and love of others. An imbalance in this chakra may manifest itself in an overwhelming feeling of disconnection from self and others. Grief, hopelessness, and inability to forgive are other manifestations of fourth chakra imbalance.

The fifth, or throat, chakra is the energy for communication and expression in our lives. When it is imbalanced or blocked, our natural self-expression is shut down, and that leads to anxiety, nervousness, and fear. I have also noticed that an imbalance of the throat chakra is often related to thyroid problems.

The sixth, or third eye, chakra is the energy center for our ability to connect with our intuition and intellectual clarity. An imbalance here leads to difficulty in thinking clearly and connecting with our intuition, which makes it hard to make decisions that are in alignment with the bigger plan for our lives.

The seventh, or crown, chakra is the energy center for our spiritual connection and divine wisdom. An imbalance here can affect the entire body.

When I was 22 years old, I met my mentor in naturopathic medicine. He was grounded and spiritual, and he often called out my lack of feminine energy. At the time, I had no idea what he meant, so I ignored it and kept moving forward with my life. It was a lesson I had to learn the hard way.

Then in my late 20s, I met a man who I ended up marrying. On paper, he was the perfect partner for me—he was interested in health, food, and helping transform the planet into a healthier place. He was also the perfect partner for me to grow into my life's work because he mirrored my masculine tendencies. Our dynamic was that I worked and "brought home the bacon," being strongly in my masculine side, while he indulged in his more creative, feminine side. It ended with me working 15-hour days, struggling to keep us afloat, and feeling unsupported and carrying the weight of the world on my shoulders.

We didn't start out with this dynamic though; at first, I was in a more feminine role while he was in a more masculine one. I was just starting my business, and he too was creating a business. Slowly but surely, our dynamic began changing. By the time we were living together, his business had started to collapse, and I assumed the role of the breadwinner.

When this shift happened, we moved away from the polarized masculine–feminine necessary for a healthy relationship. As a result, our intimacy and ability to be together declined, and we had lots of fights. Even though we weren't trying to have a baby at the time, I can see how that would also play a role in a healthy relationship. A part of me refused to have a child with him because I couldn't imagine caring for a child when I was working 15-hour days and not receiving much support in the other aspects of my life.

Though I would not choose ever to go back to that place, being there taught me a few great lessons. For one, it helped me discover my tendency to be masculine. Although it was my natural pattern to take on and do more, achieve more, and keep pushing myself, the truth is I didn't know how to be any different until I fully lived out the masculine-centric approach to life. Being forced to take on the more masculine energy in the relationship left me completely depleted. It made me look and feel 10 years older, and I realized how much I hated being in that masculine center. If I didn't monitor this tendency and get lots of support, I would easily slide back into that pattern. In the process, I learned how to become more feminine—how to embrace and embody the feminine energy. I also learned that I enjoy being in the feminine energy much more than the masculine!

Now I am much more grounded, more present in my body, and as a result, I'm more tuned into my needs and have learned to ask for and receive support. All of this is crucial for being in the feminine. Now I have a partner who embodies his masculine, which allows me to stay gracefully in my feminine so that I get to be creative and flow through life with much more ease. For that, I am very grateful, so much so that I recognize that the creative birthing of this book would have been impossible without his masculine support.

What has been most important for me to learn (and re-train my mindset) is that being in the feminine does not mean I don't run my business, work hard, or have responsibilities. Actually, it's quite the opposite. Being more in my feminine has led me to be more successful in my business. I believe it's because I have a lot more support. I have been on the receiving end of a fair amount of healing work (the kind of work I do with my clients) to shift my energy to ask for support and receive it when it is offered. The same methods also helped me release old trauma and wounds from various locations in my body. I had many deeply ingrained patterns that had to be brought to light and healed in order to create the space in my life to be more feminine. All of these things have supported my process of embracing my feminine, and I believe it is always a work in progress.

What Is Masculine and Feminine Anyway?

There are many ways to define the masculine and feminine energies. Based on the studies I have done, I would summarize them as follows: Masculine energy is penetrative and direct. It moves in a straight line and can often seem to push over or blast through the things that are in its way. It is the energy of having a goal and going for it, no matter what. On a physical level, it can be observed in the movement of sperm. Sperm move with this force and directness, driven to fertilize an egg. Feminine energy is more circular and giving. It has the capacity to turn, bend, and adapt, even if it is moving toward a goal. In the process of reproduction, the womb receives the sperm, having space for it to travel through the cervix and allowing the healthiest sperm to penetrate the egg. The feminine is more about receiving, while the masculine is more about giving or directing. Women operating from their masculine centers will be more directive, piercing, and controlling, more so than when they are operating from their feminine centers. Neither of them is good or bad, and when in balance we can call on whichever we need in any moment. The problem occurs when we are heavily situated in one and have trouble shifting into the other. We all have and need both energies within us, and we have the capacity to choose which center we operate from.

Role Reversal and Its Consequences

Without being sexist or anti-feminist, I would like to say that in the midst of the feminist movement, we might have lost the art of the feminine. In the process, we, as a culture, have emasculated men.

Masculine energy is that of a single focused provider, but how many men live in that place today? These days, there is a role reversal where more and more men are stay-at-home dads while the women are the breadwinners of the households.

Though couples may decide to let the woman take on the traditionally masculine role and the man take on the traditionally more feminine role in their household, there is a potential problem with that arrangement. If the woman spends her creative energy on running a business or generating income, she will have very little energy left over for baby creation. As a very simple explanation, the second chakra, the second energy center from the bottom, is located in the sacral area. This is the area that controls or provides the energy to be creative and construct things. If women are creating a business or investing a lot of their creative energy into their careers, it is very hard for them to have the energy left over for a thriving sex life or conceiving a baby. Is it any surprise then that it's difficult for hardworking women to have the energy to have children? The complaint I hear most often from women is that they do not have the time to cook, take care of themselves, read a book, etcetera. Being the breadwinner comes at the cost of self-care. If they don't have the time to cook a meal, how will they have the time to raise a child? Also, if the women are the breadwinners of their families, and they become mothers, they might feel like they are doing everything, which can cause a lot of frustration and fear. It's vital to make time for self-care, and doing so can be fun. It is important for women on the fertility or conception path to be centered in their feminine so that they can receive the energy of the baby and co-create this child with their partner. Even for same-sex couples, it is important for the woman who will carry the child to be more in her feminine essence.

Another frustration I hear a lot pertains to timed intercourse. If you have been on the fertility journey for a while, you know exactly what I'm talking about. It's looking at your clock and thinking, "I'm ovulating. Time to have sex!" It can be frustrating to both sexes, but I hear the complaint more often from men than women. Even though they get lots of sex, the men can feel like they are being used for their sperm, which emasculates them. Also, because sex becomes such a regimented experience, it takes away from the energy that has the potential to support the creation of a baby. The feminine turns toward the masculine, and the masculine turns toward the feminine, and this de-polarization of the energy leads to reduced sex drive for both parties. The way back is simple; it's to re-polarize the masculine and feminine.

Around the time I was struggling in the relationship with my ex-husband, I had a patient who had been trying to have a child for a long time who shared many of my struggles. She too was the breadwinner of the family. Her husband hadn't worked for several years, and she was taking care of him. The more she urged him to find a job and go back to being a caretaker, the more he felt pushed away and deprived of his masculinity.

As soon as she was able to shift back into her feminine, a transformation happened. She could relax and surrender, and he was able to find work and start supporting them again. She didn't stop working; she just shifted the way she worked and how she was at home. She went from having an aggressive attitude to a more relaxed and feminine one. She stopped trying to be in control and rather allowed things to flow. She powerfully asked for what she wanted in a feminine way—and got it! This shift allowed for a breakthrough between her and her husband. Her husband now felt less emasculated and controlled by her, and because of this shift in their energy, they were able to conceive.

Tools to Reclaim the Feminine

The first step to reclaiming the feminine is to identify if you have lost your feminine energy and your partner has lost his masculine energy. You can identify the loss of feminine energy by evaluating the number of day-to-day household chores that are on your shoulders. If your partner is spending most of his time at home doing "nothing"—watching TV, being on the computer, whatever it is—and you feel weighed down and drained from your hours of work, you don't feel supported emotionally or financially by him, and you don't have time to do anything you love, you may have lost your feminine energy. The loss of the masculine is a little bit more difficult to identify. Unless you ask him, there is no way for you to know. If he seems depressed, doesn't engage with you, and doesn't have passion or sexual energy toward you, you might want to have a conversation with him and ask if he feels emasculated or if the relationship isn't fulfilling for him. If you have assumed the masculine role of taking care of everything and supporting the household, more likely than not, your partner has assumed the feminine role. My belief is that the woman can shift the balance in one direction or the other. As soon as the woman shifts, the man tends to shift into the opposite. Just as easy as it is for the woman to shift back into the feminine, the man can shift into the masculine.

If you discover that there has been a role reversal, then the next step is to reconnect with your feminine by getting sensual. The hormone oxytocin is triggered by and triggers intimacy. "Oxytocin causes relaxation, fearlessness, bonding, and contentment,"[3] says Dr. Brizendine, author of *The Female Brain*. Cortisol blocks oxytocin and shuts off of the woman's desire for sex and physical touch abruptly. The release of oxytocin will help you reconnect with your feminine. You can increase the release of oxytocin with the following:

- Increased touch when and where appropriate
- Skin-to-skin contact on a daily basis
- Nipple stimulation
- Long hugs (each at least 20 seconds) several times a day

---

3   Brizendine, L. (2006). *The Female Brain*. New York: Broadway Books.

- Slow kissing
- Intimate conversations with your beloved or a girlfriend.

The isolation that can come from infertility leads to declining levels of oxytocin and dopamine, two of the major hormones contributing to women feeling pleasure and a sense of well-being, which is critical for fertility. So opening up and having an intimate conversation with a girlfriend can help release oxytocin as well as dopamine. It will both help you feel better and support your fertility.

Dance! Shake that booty! Put on some music and work those hips. Set aside time to play and connect with your inner child. Also, prepare your food. Not only is it much better for your health to eat homemade food, but the sight and smell of the food as you are preparing it also helps release oxytocin. Receiving massages and nesting as if your baby were already here will trick your brain into releasing oxytocin as well. Then get out of your left brain by engaging in activities you love like music, sewing, art, etcetera.

Last but not least, have orgasms with or without ovulation. You don't have to be ovulating to have great sex. Engage even if you're not trying so that you can keep the levels of oxytocin high. It will support the balance of the masculine and feminine energies in your relationship.

Expand Your View of What It Is to Be a Woman

Do you want to have an amazing career or business and still have a baby? Go ahead! You can admit it. I'm totally with you. I love what I do; at the same time, in the near future, I would like to have a child.

It's not so much *what* you do but *how* you do it that makes a difference. Could you be more feminine in the way you run your business or do your job? What would that look like? If the first picture of being more feminine that comes to your mind is to be a pushover or not to have enough clout in your company, know that this is the negative and distorted image of the feminine.

As I mentioned earlier, our culture values the masculine. Women are taught at a young age not to be "too girly" and observe men call each other derogatory names like "pussy," which send the message that being feminine is not good or valuable and should be avoided. Mama Gena's book *Pussy* captures the essence of the movement we as women need to reclaim the feminine by reclaiming the word *pussy*. Many of the practices in Mama Gena's book might support you on your path to embracing your divine feminine.

In its authenticity, the feminine has many faces: the warrior, the destroyer, the bringer of truth, the goddess, the queen, and the seductress, just to name a few. These are all ways of being that come from various mythologies. The common theme is that women have many faces, which are depictions of powers within us—facets of the divine feminine. Some of us use one power more freely than another. And some of us choose the masculine energy within us to move about our day-to-day lives.

There are many modes of the feminine, and there is no one box I want to put you in. Instead, I want to help you identify your go-tos and shift into a more expansive version of yourself that can pull out whatever manifestation you need on any given day. The empowered feminine is the woman who can be the warrior and destroyer when that is needed and then become the queen or seductress when the occasion calls for that. That is the full exploration of what is possible as a woman.

CHAPTER 4

Reclaiming the Feminine, Embracing the Cycle of Creation

The Seasons of the Month

We have many cycles in our existence—some that apply to everything and everyone on the planet including plants and animals, like the seasons, and some that are specific to us women. What's fascinating to me is that our menstrual cycle is a 28-day look into the whole of the universe. Let me show you what I mean.

Menses is the season of winter. It can be in sync with the new moon and is the darkest time of the cycle emotionally. According to the philosophy of Chinese medicine, menses is naturally our most *yin* time. It is when things are (or should be) slow. In many tribal societies and cultures, women wouldn't have to cook, clean, or do any work during this time. Instead, they would have this time to receive and be taken care of by those they supported and cared for the rest of the month. It is also a time when powerful wisdom and intuition is at its peak. If you can, consider receiving help and support during this time.

Slow down or take time off when possible, and spend your time going deep within to receive the wisdom of your soul, or at the very least, use this time to set deep intentions, whether for baby-receiving or for other things you wish to receive or transform in your life.

The time from the end of menses up to ovulation is the spring season. In this time of bloom, we are growing and developing one magical egg that will be released. If you are actively trying to get pregnant, this is a good time to send your ovaries love and attention to grow the egg to its fullest potential. It is also a good time to be more active in your life, and don't forget to stop and smell the roses!

Spring is a magical time. In this season, I have a little extra skip in my step and a lot of gratitude for being in my body and for the beauty in the world. If being in a state of gratitude is not natural to you, I invite you to create a gratitude journal. Every day, just make a list of three things you're grateful for. Look for beauty and joy in your surroundings as well as within you. Even though you may feel upset with yourself or your body for not being pregnant yet and disappointed that you had a cycle once again, try to step out of that place. The best way to shift this self-deprecating energy is with gratitude and appreciation.

Then comes summer—ovulation, which often syncs up with the full moon. It is the peak of our sexuality and sensuality. It's also our time to be most outwards in the world since it is our most *yang* time of our month. Don't force it, but if your body and cycles are in tune, this is likely the time you feel the friskiest. Sex drive goes way up because your natural state is to procreate, and this is the peak time to conceive. Give yourself love for being so in tune with your body.

If your sex drive is not elevated during this time, do things around this time that can help you get more sensual such as cooking, listening to music, laying on silky soft sheets, etcetera. See tips on how to raise oxytocin in Chapter 3. I don't recommend forcing yourself and your partner to have sex (or timing sex to your ovulation strips), though, because that often works against your ability to get pregnant. Instead, be patient with yourself and give your body time to synchronize with nature's rhythms. Trust that it will happen.

If increasing the oxytocin in your body doesn't increase your sex drive over time, I can recommend using yoni eggs, which are egg-shaped crystals with the properties of the crystals they are made of. My favorites are rose quartz eggs (helpful in increasing self-love and fertility) and jade eggs (known for improving fertility and womb health). You can purchase the yoni eggs online. Once you have procured the egg of your choice, insert it vaginally during the time between the completion of your menstrual cycle and ovulation. You can continue using it through ovulation and up till the start of your next menses if you wish. Regular use of the egg will increase your cervical mucus, which will bring more energy and flow into your reproductive organs and likely help to increase your sex drive.

Post-ovulation is the fall season, when things are colorful but slowly starting to wither away like the leaves falling from the trees. This is often the time when the unconscious becomes conscious. Our intuition is on the rise, and any discord or disharmony between our spirit and body is likely to manifest itself as PMS. PMS, which is usually blamed on the hormones, is not the same experience for everyone. Many women have no symptoms at all. If you have PMS symptoms, ask yourself what you have pushed under the rug for the whole month. Are you feeling run down and unsupported? Then you probably skimped on self-care this month. Are you feeling angry with your partner? Then you probably had some issues you chose not to voice during the month. Are you upset with your boss for giving you too much responsibility? Then it's probably time to ask for a raise. Instead of blaming your hormones for the emotional discord they are creating in your life, take a moment to pause and look at the information being presented to you. It is a great time for you to tune in and listen to what your body is telling you. When you address those things, the PMS improves and eventually goes away.

Get to Know Your Cycle

Getting to know your body and your cycle is a key step to fertility. Of the many things I teach my clients as I work with them, the tool of tracking basal body temperatures (BBTs), which are core body temperatures measured upon waking up, and understanding what the shift in these temperatures means for your fertility is probably the most essential. Start by measuring your temperature as soon as you wake up every morning.

The follicular temperatures, measured between cycle Day 1 and ovulation, of an optimal BBT chart are slightly lower than post-ovulation temperatures. The "normal" cycle chart dips slightly just before ovulation, rises during ovulation, and stays high through the luteal phase. For those who are new to fertility verbiage, your *follicular phase* is the first half of your cycle, going from Day 1 (the day you start menses) to midway of the cycle, ideally between Day 13 and 16 of your cycle. The luteal phase is the latter part of your cycle after ovulation happens and continues till the start of your next menstrual cycle.

A few temperature patterns that point to imbalance and what they might indicate are:

- Consistently low temperatures (below 97.8 F) might point to thyroid imbalance or low body temperature syndrome
- An up and down (peaks/valleys) pattern in the follicular part of the cycle indicates an imbalance in FSH (follicle stimulating hormone) or estradiol, or both
- An up and down (peaks/valleys) pattern in the luteal phase indicates malnutrition or malabsorption

- Low but consistent temperatures in the post-ovulation phase indicate low progesterone levels

- Very low temperatures in the follicular phase (that rise normally afterward) might be related to high estradiol

- A lack of a clear peak temperature might indicate anovulation

- An abnormally long cycle without a clear peak temperature might indicate polycystic ovarian syndrome

- A luteal phase less than 10 days (the number of days between peak temperature and menses) might point to low progesterone, low ovarian reserve, or poor egg quality.

As you can see, tracking basal body temperatures is valuable and almost essential. Many women tell me they hate doing it, but once they understand how much information we can gather just from looking at these temperature patterns, they are usually more willing to start doing it regularly.

When you get skilled at basal body temperature tracking, it can also serve as a viable approach to hormone-free birth control. Many studies have found BBT tracking to be a 98% effective tool for birth control if done correctly.[4,5] So if you're trying to preserve your fertility for later and want an option for natural birth control, I suggest getting some training in basal body temperatures.

---

[4]   Manhart, M.D., Duane, M., Lind, A., Sinai, L., Golden-Tevald, J. (2013). Fertility awareness-based methods of family planning: A review of effectiveness for avoiding pregnancy using SORT. *Osteopathic Family Physician*, 5(1), 2-8.

[5]   Fehring, R. J., Schneider, M., Raviele, K., & Barron, M. L. (2007). Efficacy of cervical mucus observations plus electronic hormonal fertility monitoring as a method of natural family planning. *Journal of Obstetric, Gynecologic & Neonatal Nursing*, 36(2), 152-160. doi:10.1111/j.1552-6909.2007.000129.x

The Seasons of the Day

Generally speaking, we have a mini-version of the 28-day cycle every day, which is reflected in the cortisol rhythm of the body. The night is the winter—our peak yin period to curl up in bed and sleep. The waking-up time is the spring. Our cortisol increases in the morning, giving us energy for the day. The peak yang time is mid-day, which can be thought of as summer. And the evening is the fall when things slow down and impressions of events from our day begin to wither away. Being out of sync with this daily cycle is also problematic. For example, if we skip out on our sleep time—the time to rest, rejuvenate, and receive intuition from our soul, which happens while we sleep—it turns into an out-of-balance day. For women, being out of sync with the daily cycle will often lead to being out of sync with the monthly cycle. Learning to embrace the rhythm of your day and month is crucial to having optimal hormonal balance and fertility.

Tune into the Rhythms of Your Body

There are a few things you can do to tune into the rhythms of your body and get back in sync if you feel out of it. I have adapted these universal recommendations from Christiane Northrup and applied them to the fertility journey as I have seen them play out in my patients.

1. **Be selfish.** Going along with someone else's plan for you or beating up yourself for doing something you believe is right for you but society disagrees with is going to show up as PMS. Don't do it! It just leads to discord, resentment, anger, etcetera. Do what *your* spirit and soul guide you to do.

2. **Stop trying to be perfect.** A lot of us women believe we need to be perfect in order to be loved. And we often have the idea of a perfect plan, a perfect life, and the "right" time to have a

baby—our schedule for what is perfect. Sometimes that may not be the ideal time in the life that is waiting for you.

3. **Get support.** Surround yourself with people who support and love you for who you are—people who believe in the highest good for you and want the best for you. For example, will an infertility support group support you to be your highest and best fertile self, or will it try to bring you down to get you to accept yourself as infertile? It's up to you to decide. I don't believe in any labels, but I especially don't believe in the "infertile" label. That is why this entire book focuses on how to be fertile, not on "infertility," and my advice to you is to do the same. Divorce yourself from the word *infertile* and stop being around people who label you as such. Instead find yourself in a positive and uplifting community that reaffirms your ability to become fertile.

4. **Ask for help.** Asking for help is hard for both men and women. Some women have told me they don't even know what they need help with. It goes back to listening to your intuition and tuning into your body to figure out where you need the help. Once you figure out what you need, learn to ask for the help. First and foremost, allow your husband to help you. It doesn't make you weak or less than; it actually makes him feel great! Trust me; men *love* to help. When framed correctly, he will love supporting you by doing the laundry, taking out the trash, or making you tea every night.

One of my clients does exactly that—he makes his wife tea every night, cleans, does the laundry, and more! As little as four months ago, however, he was not doing any of these things. Instead, he felt at a loss for what he could do to help his wife relax and have some down time. He is close to 50, and his wife is 42 years old. When they came to me, they had been on the fertility journey for a few years and had tried many of the conventional options offered to them. As much as my heart broke when they told me their story, I could also see how in love they were and how they had not let their journey bring them down—they were full of *joie de vivre*.

When they flew in from New York City, where they live, to the Bay Area, where I live and practice, for the hands-on component of their program, I got to spend a fair amount of time with them. As luck would have it, the woman had stopped having a period after her last IVF cycle seven months prior to meeting me. Her AMH was very low, and her FSH was high. I realized that she was extremely busy, but more importantly, I saw that she was stressed out by a feeling that she had to hold together all the pieces in her relationship; her family, including her father who had cancer; and the family business that couldn't function without her. She felt like she had to do it all herself. Interestingly enough, her body showed signs of being extremely sensitive to the slightest stress, so her capacity to handle the things life threw her way was pretty minimal. It was challenging for her to relax and let in help and support, but she needed to receive, and her husband (the sweetest man ever) was trying to be giving to her. To increase her ability to receive, I invited her to step into her feminine.

At the time that I'm writing this book, they haven't gotten pregnant yet, but her FSH is much lower than it was before they started working with me, she's cycling and ovulating normally (which in itself is a miracle!), and their chances of conceiving are much better than four months ago, so much so that even her reproductive endocrinologist is supportive of her trying naturally rather than undergoing another IVF cycle. I believe that her ability to relax and receive has been integral in restoring her periods and improving her fertility.

If you aren't sure about letting your man give to you while you receive or letting someone else be in the driver seat for once, I recommend checking out the book *The Queen's Code* by Alison Armstrong. This book has transformed my life and the lives of many women I work with, and I highly recommend it. Once you allow and receive help from your husband, tune in and see what else you need. What does your uterus need? Does your intuition tell you that you need a fertility specialist, someone to hold space for your healing so that you can get fertile and have a family? If so, find the right team of holistic practitioners. Don't wait. Trust your gut and go for it. If your intuition says that you don't need any other help, then be okay with that too. There is no "right"; just feel into your intuition (especially during your premenstrual and menstrual phases when it is at its peak) and let it lead you to your right path.

CHAPTER 5

Triumph Over Grief and Judgment

I have always been fascinated by the mind and emotions. When I was in undergraduate school, I looked for ways to take more psychology classes, and in medical school, I was fascinated by homeopathy, which addresses underlying mental–emotional concerns.

It was no surprise to me that one of my first fertility patients had an overall sad disposition even though she seemed physically healthy. It was as if she was holding on to a lot of sadness and grief. After several appointments, she finally opened up to me about how she had never properly processed the grief of having an abortion in her 20s. Although she knew it was the best decision for her at the time, she carried a lot of sorrow about it—especially since she now was having trouble conceiving. She felt as though this was her punishment for having chosen to have an abortion earlier in life.

To be able to conceive and have a healthy pregnancy, she needed to process the grief, which she did with a proper homeopathic remedy. We also needed to find the location of the grief in her body. We discovered that she housed her grief in her large intestine. Interestingly enough, she had had constipation for a good portion of her life, and when she was able to release the emotion from that region of her body, she got healthier bowel movements. Soon after she had processed the grief, and we had cleared the emotions from her body, she got pregnant.

In this chapter, we will look at the feelings that are associated with past miscarriages, abortions, and getting your period when you are trying to conceive. We will observe and get an understanding of how these deeper emotions can get stuck in your body and potentially block your ability to conceive. Then we will look at how to overcome them and triumph over judgment—from yourself as well as other people.

Feelings Associated with the Fertility Journey

People around you may have a lot of thoughts and opinions on you getting pregnant. Let's say it's the holidays, and you go home to visit your family, where one by one everyone in the family asks, "How about that baby? When are you going to have it?" Perhaps they don't know you are trying, so they are affecting you without knowing it. Or maybe they know you are trying, and they tell you what to do, what to eat, what to drink, what magic supplement to take, or even how you should feel. If you have been on this fertility journey for a year or more, I'm confident someone in your life has tried to tell you there is some magic thing that you're not doing that you should do to get pregnant.

Perhaps family and friends provide some well-intended advice: "Oh, don't worry about it; just stop trying. It will happen when you least expect it to." That might be great advice to embrace, but if you have already been trying to conceive for several years, you might be provoked by being told that it will happen on its own. It might tempt you to shut down and close off from the world to protect your heart. Though friends and family mean well, there is no magical drink or food that will help you get pregnant immediately. If there were a magic remedy, someone would be incredibly rich. Unfortunately, there is no magic, so let's take that off the table.

The comments and advice from family and friends add to the feeling of judgment that you may already have toward yourself. Under the feeling of judgment is a sense of shame: "Maybe something is wrong with me. Maybe my body can't do what every other woman's body can do." If you feel that way, let me tell you that it's an entirely normal emotion.

If that feeling causes you to close off and shut down, however, there is something you need to examine more carefully. Hold the emotion lightly, without judgment. After you have allowed yourself to hold the feeling, then, without judging it or pushing it away, breathe through it. When you are ready, let it go and invite in a more empowering perspective.

You are perfect just the way you are, even if you feel like something is wrong with you! In all my years of practice, I have never met anyone with whom there was something "wrong." One person who contacted me once was born without a uterus. Sure, that meant that she would not be able to carry a child, but that didn't mean that she was any less of a woman or that there was something wrong with her. It just meant that she would need some extra loving support.

I'm a proponent of support without the "less than" attitude. It's not for doctors or family members to make you feel like you're not good enough or that something is wrong with you. I think of it as just the way things are. When people have cancer, we don't blame them for it or make them feel like something is wrong with them because of it, right? So why are fertility issues made so personal? There is nothing the matter with you! And you are no less of a woman than you were before you started trying to have a baby.

What I have found in my practice is that many women feel negative emotions not only because of what their families or friends say to them, but also because of things that happened to them earlier in life. There could be shame from events in childhood, or there could be unprocessed grief from a miscarriage or an abortion in earlier years. I see this often my practice. On a subtler level, every time a woman who is actively trying to conceive gets her period, there is a subtle grief or disappointment. The fertility journey is a bit unique because as humans, we anticipate grieving the loss of a parent or pet, but how do you grieve something you never had? That is not commonly accepted in our culture as something to mourn. When this continues for many months, sometimes years, the grief and disappointment may accumulate.

Emotions Stuck in the Body

All these negative emotions go "undercover" and settle in certain parts of the body. It's like a protective mechanism; if you can hide away the emotions somewhere in the body, then you don't have to deal with them at the time they are happening. We know from psychology research that traumas, for example, get displaced into the subconscious and are often repressed so that they can be forgotten. Through my years of practice, I have seen that emotions can be similarly hidden in the body.

Infertility is an interesting way for the body to resurface some of the emotions that have been pushed down and not yet dealt with. For example, the uterus and ovaries are the storehouses of emotions related to our sexuality, experiences around sexuality, past abuse, how we were raised, or a parent telling us that we're ugly. When negative emotions associated with these types of things are stored in the reproductive system, it may contribute to the inability to conceive, which triggers the negative emotions and amplifies the judgment already present.

Many of the women I work with experience grief, but one woman in particular comes to mind. She came to me when she was around 38 years old, carrying a lot of grief and sadness. Already as a child, she had had a sad disposition, and now as an adult, she was even sadder. She couldn't quite put her finger on where the grief was coming from or why she was even grieving, though. There wasn't anything in particular about her life that she was sad about, and since she hadn't lost anything, she felt that she couldn't grieve. And most of the people around her had no idea that she was sad because she did a great job hiding it.

We found the emotions of sadness and grief in her ovaries and fear housed in the kidneys. As we went through the treatment, we realized that it wasn't her sadness she was carrying around all this time. Rather, it was sadness that she had inherited from her mother when she was in the womb. When I asked my client what she knew about what had happened when she was in the womb, she told me that it was the time when her father had decided to leave because he couldn't handle it anymore, and her mother had felt alone during the pregnancy with no partner or family to support her. As we dug further, we found that my client feared that once she got pregnant, her partner would leave her, though he had shown no signs of doing what her father had done.

To clear her of the sadness, we had to clear her ancestral energies. To do that, I asked the body questions and listened to what it revealed through biofeedback. Biofeedback techniques are based on the energy fields surrounding the body that allow the practitioners to ask yes or no questions to the clients and receive the clients' body–mind wisdom. The biofeedback allowed us to access the intuition of the client and uncover the deeper issues in an organic way. It is very much an integrated mind¬–body approach. Sure enough, two weeks after we had completed her treatment, she got pregnant.

Overcoming the Emotions

Even though I can't provide scientific proof for it, it is a common experience that clearing deep emotions such as grief, fear, judgment, and shame out of your body can remove the blocks to your fertility. To release the emotions and make space for a healthy pregnancy, it's imperative to discover where the emotions are hidden. If you want to transform your emotions on your own, it will be up to you to find out where your body is storing them and release them. Deep breathing and meditation can often help uncover these emotions. Call on your intuition to guide you. If you are willing to get the support of someone who can help uncover the stuck emotions and release them from your body, you might find that the process goes faster. I know that when I have stuck emotions, it's easier for me to get unstuck when I have someone who can hold a neutral space to discover what is stuck and intuitively guide my body in the way that it chooses to process and release those emotions. For each person, this process might be different. The way I practice, there is no one-size-fits-all but rather a deep listening to the client's body to help discover what is ready to be released and healed.

Once you have found and released the emotions of grief, sadness, fear, anger, judgment, or resentment (whatever it is that is in the way of you and a family), you can replace them with empowering beliefs. For example, it could be the belief that your body has the ability to heal itself, to rebalance and conceive a healthy baby, or that you are in alignment with your spirit and can surrender to whatever needs to happen on your life path. You know your body well. It has the ability to do what is natural for it to do. Every day, you feed that belief or hack away at it. You have that choice. My suggestion is to feed it. I believe our bodies are capable of reproducing if they are given all the right nutrients and support they need. Fertility is a complex issue; hence the solution is always going to be complex. It needs to take into account you as an individual and the underlying cause or challenges. No path you are on should discredit your ability to know what is happening in your body and take away your trust that what you're experiencing is your truth. You should not feel shame or judgment about having difficulty becoming pregnant. Remember, those sentiments can become blocks. It is also important to not allow other people to impose their judgments or shame for you onto you. Do not take on other people's thoughts! It's your choice whether or not you have the belief in your own body. My suggestion is that you empower and reiterate that belief in your body as much as you can. If you notice blocks, grief, or judgment coming, then look for the root of the feeling, determine where it's stuck in your body, and get it out. Don't reinforce it and let other people retrigger the emotion in you.

It's often hard to let family or friends know when they are not supporting you in your journey. I want to encourage you to openly share whatever you feel like sharing. If someone responds to you by telling you that you're not doing something that would magically help you get pregnant, tell that person that is not supportive and that it's making you feel whatever it is you're feeling at the moment. Be honest and truly think about it. Re-acknowledge to yourself that you know your body best, and follow your heart and spirit.

CHAPTER 6

Healing Is Not Curing

Let's take a moment to look at healing versus curing. When people have infections and take antibiotics that make their symptoms go away, they are considered cured by the standards of Western medicine. And when people with diabetes have lower blood sugar levels, they no longer have the symptoms and are considered cured as long as they continue their medications. In either of these cases, are people healed?

In this chapter, I want to discuss the misperception many people have around curing and disease. Western medicine aims for curing, which means removing the symptoms. Eastern medicine aims for healing, which is symptom relief on a deeper level achieved in a gentler way that doesn't suppress the disease further. Health is not merely the lack of disease; it is also a state of inner freedom—freedom to grow, evolve, and develop in order to manifest your highest potential. Health is also harmony with nature, a state in which you can listen to the voice within. Dis-ease is the lack of ease in the body. It may be defined as a state that is not conducive to the inner harmony or further evolution of people. It is an energetic imbalance and a shift in our natural vitality that is not beneficial. The disease state is usually not just on one level such as the most commonly associated physical symptoms, whether it be pain, heart disease, ulcers, etcetera. There are underlying mental, emotional, and spiritual components with every imbalance, be it a toothache, heart disease, or cancer. The physical symptoms are usually the last manifestations of many other underlying imbalances.

Disease is like growing weeds in a beautiful garden. The weeds may grow for various reasons. A cure is like the removal of the weeds. The weeds may grow back just as easily as they came—if not in the same location then another, if not the same weeds then some others. The weeds will be in the beautiful garden until the *cause* of them is removed. The removal of the cause is healing. Mere removal of the symptoms or weeds is what has been called curing. Although this will bring some relief to the patient, the disease may manifest in a new way or somewhere else in the body.

Let's consider a patient with ovarian cancer for example. The patient is advised to get a hysterectomy as a cure. She undergoes the surgery plus the additional chemotherapy and radiation she has been recommended. Five years later, the patient is diagnosed with breast cancer. Why? Because curing does not equal healing. Like the weeds in the garden, the root cause of the disease has to be removed or altered for healing to occur. With the patient, removing the uterus and ovaries in the hysterectomy didn't remove the problem. A lot of Western doctors might look at that and say, "Well, it's not the same disease. It's breast cancer now, not ovarian or uterine cancer." Yes, the location has changed. Even the disease process—the way the cells are growing—might be different. At the very core of the disease, however, it is the same energetic pattern that keeps repeating itself.

The negative patterns have to be reversed back to positive ones for a person to become truly healthy. In my practice, I always aim to heal by shifting the patterns not conducive to health and bringing balance to my patients' state of being, not cure. My patients are active participants in their processes and journeys. I'm only there as a guide on their journeys. We all have within us what we need in order to heal, but it often takes another person to lead the way to healing and health. Aim for true healing, not just curing the problem!

Naturopathic medicine encompasses many modalities, which means it offers a lot of tools to aid the healing process. I use several modalities throughout my patients' fertility journeys, and I want to share them with you—not because you need to look into each one but to widen your perspective regarding what healing modalities are available to you. You may or may not already have tried some of them.

Homeopathy

Homeopathy is the first modality I will cover because it's the most debated. I believe in science. I also believe in the "woo" (my word for the non-scientific, more energy-based approaches to healing). Most of all, I believe in anything I can use to support the healing processes of my clients. Many people consider homeopathy to be placebo and hence, ineffective. Though I may be inclined to agree, I have seen the value of appropriate homeopathic remedies given at the appropriate times, and I have found it to be tremendously supportive and transformative for my patients.

Homeopathy is an energetic healing mechanism and system that takes into account the whole person based on the principles of like cures. The purpose of homeopathy is to bring into alignment non-beneficial patterns of energy, whether they may be physical, mental or emotional. Homeopathic practitioners spend time questioning the patients to ascertain their energy so that it can be matched with the energy of the remedy. The process of question and answer alone can be very healing, bringing the patients' patterns or imbalances to the forefront gently.

In addition, homeopathic remedies are used to align patients' energies to work for them rather than against them. With the appropriate homeopathic remedies, the patients' energies begin working for them as intended by nature so that the healing of their minds, bodies, and spirits can occur without being blocked by the impediments they have put up.

What makes homeopathy difficult to understand is that it's the exact opposite of Western medicine, where the medicine is stronger the higher the dosage of the medicine is. The best way to understand homeopathy is to relate it to the idea of vaccines. Though homeopathic remedies are not vaccines, they, like vaccines, are diluted substances that help to heal. As homeopathic remedies are energy, the more diluted they are from their physical state, the stronger they become. When patients receive the correct treatment, amazing things can happen!

In an earlier chapter, I shared with you the story of one of my clients who thrived on control. She was 40 years old, had been through several IVF cycles, and had been struggling with infertility for about five years. She was quite unaware of her need for control, but since she was willing to do anything to have a child, at one point, I broached the topic. I said, "Listen, I think your need to be in control is getting in the way of your fertility."

"What do you mean, control?" she replied.

"Well, you have expressed how much you like telling your husband what to do and what not to do. I haven't talked to him, but surely, he feels controlled. Then I noticed that your house is all white and super clean. How do you think a child will respond to that environment?"

Her first reaction was to defend the way she lived, but as she was talking, she realized that control was one of the main issues of her life. When we got to the root of it, she said that it had started in her childhood and was a response to her upbringing. Her highly functional and sociable alcoholic, overachieving father and absentee mother had contributed to the amount of control she felt like she needed to have in her life. She was brought up to get straight A's and be the "good girl." She combined the need for control and managing others with her super achieving personality and desire to please and be successful for approval.

I gave her a homeopathic remedy based on everything she had presented, and about two weeks later, she became pregnant. Of course, there were other things we did along the way, but the homeopathic remedy helped her shift the pattern of control. Her husband later called me to see if I would give him gallon of the homeopathic remedy, just in case she ever went back to being the controlling, bossy, type-A person she had been.

Ayurveda

Ayurveda is a system for health used for centuries in the Orient. The Ayurvedic philosophy (as well as Chinese medicine) holds that there are energy channels in the body. Disease generally arises from a blockage or improper flow in one of these channels. In this form of treatment, practitioners use a special pulse and tongue diagnosis to ascertain the function or malfunction of these channels and identify the root causes of the patients' imbalances, disorders, or diseases. Once the practitioners have made the diagnoses, they can recommend appropriate herbs, diets, massages, detoxification, etcetera, to help recreate balance in the patients' bodies for optimal well-being.

Ayurveda recognizes that there are three main *doshas* in the body. Doshas are biological energies found innately within the body and mind. Each person has all three types in different proportions at birth. The specific proportions make up a person's constitution and characterize his or her body type and emotional and physical tendencies. An imbalance can lead to different disturbances or diseases in the body. Ayurvedic philosophy suggests that bringing the dosha into balance is a way to longevity and long-term health.

The main body types or doshas are Vata, Pitta, and Kapha, and there are also combinations of each of these. Ayurveda recommends specific lifestyles for each body type that will help bring the body back into balance.

In general, Vata reflects the elements of space and air. In balance, people of this body type are quick thinking, fast moving, and generally of a thin physique. They are also more prone to lose or misplace things, be less grounded, and get easily distracted. They have lots of energy for short periods of time but can get burnt out easily. Our culture drives people to be on the go and can cause imbalances in this body type. Symptoms of constipation, gas, bloating, joint pains, or anxiety can be signs of imbalance in the Vata dosha. This dosha can be kept in balance by regular meal times, wake-up and sleep times, and routines that are kept consistent from day to day. If you are this body type, take care not to burn out, get lots of rest, and make sure your digestion stays optimal with daily bowel movements and free of gas and bloating.

Pitta reflects the qualities of the element of fire. People of this body type will have strong motivation, direction, and purpose in life. They are generally sharp, with a fiery edge. Out of balance, pitta types may be quick to anger and prone to digestive disorders of diarrhea and sleep disorders of insomnia. If you are this body type, you can remain in balance by staying away from spicy foods, not skipping meals, and surrendering to the flow of life.

Kapha reflects the qualities of earth and water. Kapha types are generally easy-going, laid-back, and family oriented. Out of balance, however, Kapha types may have a tendency to overeat and could be overweight. They may also be lethargic and prone to oversleeping, and have sluggish bowel movements. Keeping Kapha in balance involves daily movement and activity, eating minimal amounts of fatty foods, and using warming herbs in the diet.

As you can see, each body type has its own characteristics and is brought into balance with different approaches. Whether it's a diet, detoxification or the use of herbs, the treatment has to take into account not only the condition but also the body type, so it has to be tailored to each person. Please note that though some herbs may be recommended for certain conditions, they may not be beneficial for your dosha (body type).

I utilize Ayurveda in the treatments of my patients. I use diet and detoxification as ways to decrease the imbalances in my clients' doshas and help them regain balance in their body types. In addition, I use traditional Western herbs by incorporating their inherent energies into the formulas that are most conducive to the patients' particular body types.

Nutrition

Nutrition is a word that comes up often. It reminds many people of protein bars and supplements. This is not nutrition. Although supplements and such can be of assistance, there is much more to an optimal diet. Nutrition is the art of viewing food as the source of well-being and health. If food is health, should it not be pure? Hormones and pesticides are added to most widely available food, which negates the food's benefits. Additionally, the overconsumption of processed food high in sugar, salt, and unnatural substances is detrimental to the body.

Instead of using food to promote health, our society has begun using it for reaching goals—usually goals to make our bodies more "perfect." The word *diet* is often associated with a short-term change to obtain a specific goal. Many people will eat a certain way until they get the results they want, and then they will go back to eating the way they used to. The next new diet comes with its particular bars, shakes, and supplements, and is said to be capable of curing disease or supporting weight loss. The Paleo diet, GAPS diet, and South Beach diet are examples of this.

Some of these diets work well for the general population because they eliminate the intake of processed foods and unhealthy fats, and increase the intake of fiber, but they are not for everyone and not for every condition. For example, the Paleo diet is currently considered the ideal diet for a lot of people, but I have experienced otherwise. I had a patient who had begun following the classic Paleo diet and came to see me because she wanted to lose 30 pounds. She was heavy-set, but her weight was a result of inflammation. We tested her food sensitivities, and sure enough, she was sensitive to all the foods she was eating in high amounts (chicken, beef, and kale).

So don't just jump on the next bandwagon! Consider getting tested and learning your body type so that you can know how best to tailor your diet to your body type and modify your eating patterns for health and fertility. This falls to the wayside when one diet is recommended for everyone. If you choose a Paleo diet, at least modify it so that it fits your Ayurveda dosha. We will go more in depth about lab testing in Chapter 11, so keep reading.

The other key aspect of nutrition is food preparation. Food should be prepared in a way that makes it easy for the body to assimilate it. Then it becomes a rich source of nutrients and supports optimal health and well-being. I advise my fertility patients to prepare their own food. The patients who take the time out of their schedules to prepare their food are the ones who do exceedingly well because they get insight into what goes into their food. Also, when you prepare food, you indulge your senses, which causes your body to release the hormone oxytocin. Oxytocin functions as a sensuality and sexuality hormone and helps you feel great. Start exploring how you might get more involved in your food preparation.

One of the most important issues for a majority of my patients is the lack of water intake. I have found that most of my patients are dehydrated. Though water is not technically part of a diet, it constitutes about 70% of the body. It is essential for moving around hormones as they are needed for signaling in the body. Water is also essential for transporting nutrients. Most importantly, the ovaries are mostly fluid and need water so they do not shrivel up. Although there may not be studies about this yet, my experience is that the ovaries need water to sustain their optimal function.

How to individualize your water intake: Each day, you need to drink at least half your body weight in ounces. In other words, if you weigh 100 pounds, you should drink 50 ounces of water per day. In addition to that personal baseline, add four cups of water for every eight-ounce cup of coffee and two cups of water for every cup of tea, whether it's caffeinated or non-caffeinated. That is your ideal amount of water intake. It may be a daunting amount of water compared to what you are currently consuming, so start slowly. It's a process.

Hydrotherapy

Another modality I use and recommend often is hydrotherapy. Hydrotherapy is the use of water for the purpose of healing. Water contains vital energy or life force, also called *prana* or *chi*, which can help the body heal when it is channeled correctly. There are many therapies that fall into nature-cure or hydrotherapy. Wet sheet packs, constitutional hydrotherapy, and internal baths all work to stimulate the body's internal prana or vital life force, assisting the healing process. I have put together a few of my favorite hydrotherapies for fertility in the *DIY Fertility Hacks* e-book that you can download for free. The e-book contains my three favorite home remedies and talks about which tool is appropriate at what time: castor oil packs (the all-time favorite way that nature-cure doctors used to support a gentle ridding of toxins from the body), vaginal steams (a very localized tissue healing for the female genitalia), and magic socks (a great way to tonify and support the immune system).

Fasting

Fasting is abstaining from foods for certain periods of time to allow the body to cleanse and detoxify and give the digestive system some much-needed rest. Many say that fasting at least one day per week is beneficial. The body accumulates toxins from food, the environment, imbalanced thoughts, and emotions. During fasting periods, the body can release these toxins. Hydrotherapy can assist this detoxification further, as it increases the body's ability to release toxins. Another way to increase the body's capacity to release accumulated toxins and debris is massage. While helpful and effective for short periods of time, fasting unsupervised for long periods of time is not recommended. Please work with a physician or trained practitioner who can help you with the detoxification process.

In addition to fasting for periods of time, there is also a new emergence of *intermittent fasting*. The suggestions for intermittent fasting are to have 12 to 16 hours without eating in a 24-hour period. This has been shown to increase weight loss and decrease inflammation.[6] Most of the research about intermittent fasting that is currently available pertains to men. For women, the general approach to intermittent fasting needs to be slightly modified. Studies found that when female rats did two weeks of intermittent fasting, their ovaries

---

[6]   Sheperd, B. (n.d). *The Benefits of Intermittent Fasting*. Retrieved August 02, 2017, from https://draxe.com/intermittent-fasting-benefits/

shrank and their menstrual cycles discontinued.[7] Unfortunately, there are not many studies on humans to base recommendations on. Dr. Amy Shah, M.D., suggests that women do intermittent crescendo fasting—intermittent fasting on two to three nonconsecutive days per week. Dr. Shah says this has less of an impact on the hormones and hunger signals that cause women to overeat or binge-eat.[8] More research is still needed on intermittent fasting, but it seems like a potentially useful modality for some women.

BodyTalk

The last modality I will discuss here is BodyTalk. BodyTalk is a biofeedback-based system that helps practitioners get to the root causes of infertility, especially when they are related to emotions stuck in different parts of the body or different belief systems stuck in the body–mind.

Since the BodyTalk is less known, I want to expound a little more about what it is. The BodyTalk System is one of the few healing systems that enables the practitioners to get feedback directly from the clients' innate wisdom to help understand what is out of balance, and then use tools that connect the body–mind to intentional healing. It is also one of the few systems that can help the body move from fight-or-flight mode into healing mode.

The BodyTalk System goes beyond the presenting symptoms and allows me to uncover the underlying story. Bringing the story into

---

[7] Kumar, S., & Kaur, G. (2013). Intermittent Fasting Dietary Restriction Regimen Negatively Influences Reproduction in Young Rats: A Study of Hypothalamo-Hypophysial-Gonadal Axis. *PLoS ONE*, 8(1). doi:10.1371/journal.pone.0052416

[8] Shah, A. (n.d.). *The Secret to Intermittent Fasting for Women*. Retrieved July 24, 2017, from https://draxe.com/intermittent-fasting-women/

consciousness can cause miraculous things to happen. My clients get profound "a-ha" moments, symptoms dissolve, and deep healing occurs. It is comprehensive, effective, and safe. It is one of the only modalities that doesn't impose a healing protocol on the body, but instead listens to the body and clear the way for the body to heal itself. It doesn't assume that the body wants to heal in a certain way, because each body-mind is different, and the path to reach a healthier state is vastly different for each individual.

General Recommendations

As I have detailed throughout this chapter, there are many ways to improve the state of your body, mind, and spirit. Keep in mind that the objective is not just curing, which can be short-term and only addresses the symptoms at hand, but healing through identifying and addressing the root cause.

From all my years of experience, training, and self-experimentation, I offer the following suggestions for optimal health and vitality:

1. Follow a diet that works for you. If you don't know what that is, find an *unbiased* expert to help you choose. (I say unbiased here because most practitioners have their own philosophies on food that they try to impose on to others. I find that it does not work like that. People's different genetic and lifestyle predispositions create different needs. So you need a practitioner who can customize your diet for you as an individual.) In general, a diet free from processed foods, non-organic foods, and sugar is optimal for almost everyone.

2. Get good sleep, and make sure you get enough sleep for your body type. In Ayurveda, the typing system clarifies how much sleep each person needs. Kapha types need at least six hours, Vata types need eight to nine, and Pitta types need something

in the middle. If you don't know which type you are, you can take a quiz online to find out. You can also just ask yourself if you feel rested when you wake up in the morning. If you don't, you are not getting the optimal amount or quality of sleep.

3. Find ways to increase stress resilience. Since we live in societies where chronic stress is unlikely to decrease, the best we can do for ourselves is to learn how to adapt and train our bodies to be less susceptible to stress.

4. Listen to your body from the beginning. It knows and shows you signs when it's starting to get wacky. Pay attention and learn your signals. Usually, the initial signs and signals get ignored, which leads to bigger signs that take longer to heal.

5. Drink lots of pure water. The mistake that many people make is to count all liquids as water intake. Your body can only absorb pure water free of chemicals, heavy metals, and sugars. So consider giving your body what's easiest for it to absorb and utilize. Sodas, teas, and coffees are dehydrating and have the opposite effect on your body. If you don't like the taste of pure water, adding fruit or a slice of lemon can make it taste delicious. Another note on water: *Do not* drink cold water or ice water. This has a negative impact on your body. Instead, drink your water at room temperature or even heated to help your digestion and metabolism as well as your core body temperature.

CHAPTER 7

Polycystic Ovarian Syndrome

Many women with infertility have no idea why they are not getting pregnant. They continue trying different approaches and don't understand why it isn't happening, which can be extremely frustrating!

One of the first steps in taking charge of your fertility is discovering and understanding the root cause. When patients come to see me, they often ask, "Why am I not getting pregnant?" Can you help me figure out this mystery?" When we identify the *why*—the underlying root cause—we know what is happening in their bodies, which helps us determine the appropriate treatment plan to increase their chances of conceiving.

A dear friend of mine often complained about symptoms of a digestive issue. She experienced gas, bloating, and indigestion, and she also had very irregular periods that followed severe PMS and other symptoms. As she was working with various practitioners over the years, I never mentioned to her that she should consider seeing me. Eventually, she asked if I could help her with her health because she wanted to look into her fertility and see how much time she had left on her clock so she could plan it out. She came to my office, and we reviewed her symptoms and did a few hormonal tests. Then we discovered that she had something called Polycystic Ovarian Syndrome (PCOS). It is a complex syndrome with many imbalances in the body at the same time. Even though she didn't have many of the typical symptoms, she had had irregular periods her entire life, and when she was not on birth control, she had PMS and irregular menstrual cycles. These are sometimes the only symptoms of PCOS.

We started treating the PCOS to help get her fertility on track early on and relieve her symptoms so she can lead a happier, healthier life until she is ready to start a family. Understanding that it was PCOS that was causing her body not to release an egg every month made her feel more in charge of her body and hormones. Now that she is aware of her condition, she can be more in control of her menstrual cycles and prepare for fertility in a very different way than if she had remained unaware.

A Widespread but Often Overlooked Problem

PCOS is quite common. Ten percent of women within reproductive age have the syndrome, and one out of every two women who has it is likely to have infertility, so understanding the symptoms early on is key. Most of the women who have the condition have had it from their teenage years.

Though PCOS is common, many of the women who have the syndrome are never diagnosed. If they have irregular periods, doctors often just prescribe birth control pills to help them get regular and don't deal with the actual problem. About half of the women who walk into my office who are diagnosed as infertile have never even been screened for it, but many of the women who have been diagnosed with infertility have this syndrome.

Common Symptoms

PCOS is a challenging disease to diagnose because it often doesn't have a lot of signs and symptoms. The syndrome might only manifest itself in irregular menstrual cycles or PMS, which may seem like normal things that you just learn to deal with. Especially if you have had it since the onset of your menstruation, you may think it's normal. But the truth is that you shouldn't have difficulties with your menstrual cycles. In the ideal state, you have no PMS, breast tenderness, bloating, or cramps. If you have these symptoms, it's important that you get checked. If you're young, don't suppress the symptoms with birth control, which may create a more severe issue that can cause infertility. Rather, treat it holistically.

As I mentioned earlier, with PCOS, there are many imbalances in the body at the same time. There are many potential signs and symptoms of the syndrome, which can relate to the following underlying imbalances:

1. Hyperandrogenism, excessive testosterone in the body, which can cause symptoms like male pattern baldness, loss of breast tissue, and growth of facial hair or excessive hair growth anywhere on the body.

2. Cysts on the ovaries that lead to and/or contribute to hormonal irregularities.

3. Anovulation, which makes it challenging to get pregnant.

4. Obesity, which may be caused by insulin dysregulation, meaning the insulin levels are going up and down, and the body doesn't have a way to regulate it or has created resistance to it, which is called insulin resistance.

Obesity used to be considered a main indicator of PCOS, but many of the women who have PCOS are not obese, so it is no longer thought that women have to be obese to have PCOS. You may have the syndrome even if you're skinny, and to determine whether or not you have it, you must be screened with some specific lab tests.

Holistic Treatment Options

If you are diagnosed with PCOS, you can be treated in a holistic way that has a high success rate of helping women conceive. The Western medicine that is most often prescribed to women who have been diagnosed with PCOS and are trying to conceive are Femara, Clomid, and Metformin. These are all designed to help with ovulation. There have been studies comparing all three of these to other, natural substances. One of those substances is Myo-Inositol, which has a 40% higher success rate in causing ovulation and rebalancing hormone levels in women with PCOS who are actively trying to conceive, hence increasing their likelihood of conception. Myo-Inositol doesn't work for all women but should be tried before going to Femara or Clomid. Metformin is used effectively to reduce insulin resistance, so it has been thought that it can be supportive for women with PCOS. Since insulin resistance is one of the main issues of PCOS, regulating blood sugar and insulin levels is imperative to the treatment of PCOS. The natural substance in N-Acetylcysteine (or NAC for short) has, however, been demonstrated to have better results than Metformin in women with insulin resistance and be more supportive of fertility.

It's key that you, with the support of a doctor, discover the root cause of your difficulty getting pregnant. When you know the root cause, you can get more specific in your treatment plan. If you have any of the symptoms I mentioned in this chapter, it's paramount that you ask your doctor to screen you for PCOS. If you are diagnosed with

PCOS, you can seek treatment from a naturopathic doctor because many natural nutrients and herbs have been demonstrated to be very effective in treating PCOS and even helping to increase conception rates. Talk to your doctor about what would best support treatment of PCOS and increase your fertility.

CHAPTER 8

Thyroid Health

You want to have a healthy baby, and you want to feel great in the process; however, you might have been trying unsuccessfully for a while and not know why it's not happening. Also, maybe your hormones have gone haywire, and you don't feel great, but you are not sure why because you have felt this way for the last 15 years. Feeling tired all the time, being cold often, losing hair, or having dry skin could all be signs of thyroid dysfunction. Thyroid health is likely a key factor for having a healthy baby as well as feeling great in your body.

I had a patient a few years ago who, at the age of 27, had already had depression, anxiety, chronic fatigue, and Fibromyalgia, which is chronic pain, for 10 years. She came to me because she was feeling out of whack, and none of the many doctors she had been to could help her determine why she was feeling that way. The first couple of years we worked together, we focused on nutrition and lifestyle. She experienced some improvements but nothing major. Then we tested her thyroid, and all of her thyroid hormone levels were normal. Not giving up, I decided to look further into her thyroid by studying her body temperature. Sure enough, it was in the mid to high 96s for a majority of the day, which is extremely low, so we decided to follow the Wilson's Low Body Temperature Protocol to elevate it. This protocol involves the rapid cycling of thyroid hormone to jumpstart a sluggish thyroid into action. I liken it to using electric shock (defibrillation) to reset normal heart rhythm. It's not quite as severe or dramatic, but it's a similar approach for resetting natural thyroid rhythm. After following Wilson's Protocol, my patient's temperatures improved and her symptoms began to go away. We had to follow up with a couple of rounds of treatment, but by the end, her mood had improved significantly, and she had more energy and almost no pain in her body.

This patient inspired me to take a closer look at optimized thyroid levels on all my patients. I also look at their body temperatures and work to bring those into the range that is optimal for fertility. I have found that optimizing my patients' thyroid hormone levels and getting their body temperatures closer to the ideal have helped them feel healthier and have healthier babies.

A lot of research suggests that sub-optimal thyroid function leads to less-than-optimal brain development of the babies when they are in the womb, but there is little to no research on the effect sub-optimal thyroid function has on fertility. Functional doctors such as myself, however, agree that a thyroid-stimulating hormone (TSH) level of 1 to 1.5 is optimal for fertility. I would add that consistently low temperatures of less than 97.8 are not supportive of optimal fertility. If you are cold all the time, you probably have a low body temperature. With low body temperatures and insufficient blood flow and circulation to the uterus and ovaries, it is harder to make the body function as an incubator. Early stage miscarriage can often be related to thyroid hormone dysfunction or sub-optimal thyroid function. You want your body temperature to be at optimal levels so that the embryo within you can grow at a healthy and normal pace.

Unfortunately, most doctors will only pay attention to the thyroid *after* you have gotten pregnant. If you are trying to conceive, then your doctor will most likely tell you that your thyroid level or TSH is normal. I have plenty of patients who come in with a TSH of 2, 2.5, or even 3, who have been told that their thyroid is functioning normally. Technically it is because the "normal" range of TSH is 0.45 to 4.5, but this is a very broad range. It tells you almost nothing about how your thyroid is actually functioning.

The Physiology of the Thyroid Hormones

To give you an understanding of the purpose of knowing these numbers, let me explain the physiology of the thyroid hormones. The pituitary in your brain releases the TSH to urge the thyroid gland to produce thyroid hormones. The TSH regulates the release of thyroid hormones from the thyroid gland. The thyroid then produces T4, which are inactive thyroid hormones, and T3, which are active thyroid hormones. In most cases, though, T4 is converted into T3 and reverse T3. Reverse T3 is a bit of an unknown, as doctors don't know quite what it does in the body yet. We do know, though, that it's likely not a good thing to have too much of it. My observation and studies demonstrate that a high reverse T3 means there are likely nutritional deficiencies getting in the way of conversion to active T3. Not enough active T3 means the body will not have optimal thyroid function, but it also means the ovaries will not have optimal thyroid function!

The body tries to self-regulate. All the hormones in the body work and regulate via negative feedback loops. When the body has enough of a particular hormone, that same hormone goes back and tells the pituitary to stop producing the signaling compound that initiates the production chain. T4 and T3 signal back with the negative feedback loop to the pituitary, alerting that enough T3 and T4 are being produced and that the thyroid doesn't need any more signaling to produce more thyroid hormones.

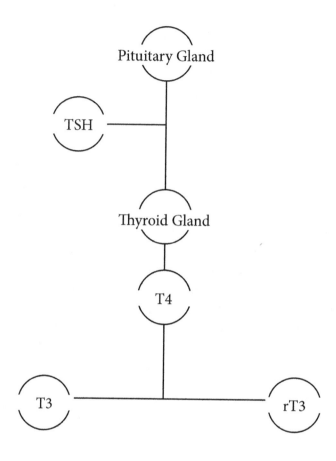

Now, say you have enough thyroid stimulating hormone, but your thyroid doesn't respond the way it should to the signaling compound. Then it won't produce T4, and there will be no feedback loop to stop the production of TSH. If the feedback never happens, the pituitary will keep putting out more TSH, and the number you would measure on a blood test would keep increasing. This is the classic definition of hypothyroidism.

There are many nuances here, though. If your body produces TSH, and your thyroid produces T4, but the T4 never gets converted to active T3, then your body doesn't have the hormone it needs to function. The signals (the T4) will then go back and signal the pituitary to stop producing TSH. As a result, the TSH number may never go up, as it would in a typical hypothyroidism condition. Unfortunately, you won't discover this conversion issue because the TSH will likely remain normal. It is one of the reasons it's paramount to have all these hormones tested from the beginning.

Thyroid Antibodies

The other aspect to understand about the thyroid is the antibodies. The antibodies are thyroglobulin antibodies (TGA), thyroid-stimulating immunoglobulin (TSI), and thyroid peroxidase antibodies (TPO). Let's say your system is producing antibodies to your thyroid. In this scenario, you may have normal levels of TSH, but your thyroid is under attack. Hence, it doesn't produce the number of thyroid hormones it would in its active form.

Thyroid antibodies are another major reason for miscarriage. Your immune system is meant to protect you from outside invaders, but sometimes that immune function goes a little haywire and starts attacking things inside your body that it should not. If your immune system is attacking your thyroid, it sees it as a foreign object. When you have antibodies to your gland or hormones, your immune system is over-activated and will go full-force at anything it views as a foreign body. If you do have these antibodies, your immune system could be attacking the embryo the same way it attacks the thyroid, and this could potentially lead to miscarriage.

As you can tell, though your doctor may consider TSH the only necessary hormone to test, there are quite a few other hormones that need to be tested to fully understand the function of the thyroid.

Your Thyroid Health

The most common early signs and symptoms of a malfunctioning thyroid gland are being colder than people around you, hair loss, fatigue, and potentially anxiety or depression. As the thyroid dysfunction progresses and continues for years, the TSH will increase if you are becoming hypothyroid or decrease if you are becoming hyperthyroid.

If you have been trying to get pregnant for a while, and you suspect you don't have an optimal thyroid hormone level, you should have all your thyroid hormones checked. It's important to have a complete panel of thyroid hormones. You wouldn't believe how many patients have come to me with just their TSH checked and been informed by their doctors that their thyroid is completely normal. Interestingly enough, TSH isn't even produced by the thyroid; it's created higher up in the chain of hormones. The changes in lab values of TSH are extremely delayed the majority of the time, so it is not the best way to catch early dysfunction of the thyroid. Other hormones are more likely to show a change in earlier stages of the problem. By measuring these, you can get to the problem faster and understand if your thyroid is playing a key role in your inability to conceive or, more commonly, carry a pregnancy to term.

In addition to all the major thyroid hormones you want to get tested (TSH, T3, free T3, T4, and reverse T3), you also want to get the three major thyroid antibodies (TGA, TSI, and TPO) tested. If you have these antibodies, you need to work on some of the underlying causes for having them. Your immune system is not working as it should be, and it needs to be addressed and healed before you try to conceive.

There are more and more studies on the thyroid hormones' effects on sperm quality and quantity. We don't normally assume that men have thyroid issues, so it's not customary to test men for this, but it's becoming increasingly more apparent that the thyroid plays a role in optimal testosterone levels and healthy sperm production. Hypothyroidism in men results in higher levels of a hormone called prolactin, which leads to lower testosterone levels and sperm production decreased to a third of its normal quantities. If your partner has low sperm counts, it's a good idea to get his thyroid levels tested as well.

The "Cheat Sheet for Understanding Your Results" guide, which you will find in the free download *Fertility Secrets Bonus Kit*, lists all the essential lab tests for fertility (including thyroid hormones) that you can use to find optimal ranges for fertility.

Even if your thyroid hormone levels are normal, if you feel tired all the time and don't have the energy to do the things you want; have anxiety, depression, chronic fatigue, chronic pain, hair loss, or dry skin; or are often cold, you are displaying signs of a potentially affected thyroid. The thyroid hormones control your metabolism and body temperature, so analysis of your body temperature is a great way to understand what is happening in its functional form and identify if your thyroid needs support, even if your thyroid hormone tests are all within normal limits. You would likely benefit from working with a holistic doctor, who can guide your analysis of your body temperatures to assess the thyroid from a functional perspective, determine the root of the issue, help figure out if your thyroid is not functioning at its optimal level, and help you get it to where it should be.

CHAPTER 9

Adrenal Health

Many women who are trying to get pregnant but haven't been able to are told by their families, "Relax, and you'll get pregnant. Just relax." Though it doesn't work exactly like that, the stress of life may affect your ability to get pregnant. Being stressed out by the fact that you're not getting pregnant can also contribute. Of course, most couples would like to go through the fertility experience with the least amount of stress possible.

When I was in medical school, I would often sigh, and my classmates would ask, "What was that for? What are you stressed out about?" My response would be, "I'm not stressed." Years after finishing med school, I went to live in a monastery for a while where I got off the grid. I would meditate many hours per day and then indulge in reading and gardening for the rest of the time. It allowed me a break from the usual pattern of being on the go. Also, after experiencing this stress-free life in the monastery, where there was incredibly clean air to breathe; pure, toxin-free water to drink; and organic, non-GMO food to eat, I realized that from the time I had started high school all the way through medical school, a continuous 12-year period, I had been stressed out without realizing it. It allowed me to recalibrate what I call my stress-o-meter so that I could take better care of myself. I can't say that I live a completely stress-free life now, but my experience at the monastery, followed by years of brain retraining and supporting the healing of my adrenal glands with herbs and supplements, I believe I am in a healthier and more balanced place.

The Impact of Stress

There are many types of stress. There is good stress, like that of having a baby on the way, and there is bad stress, like an unhappy work situation. Stress is a part of life. Even our environment and the food we eat can be stressors for the body. In Chapter 12, we will discuss the many environmental stressors that our bodies have to process.

For a more nuanced understanding of stress, you need to comprehend how the body experiences the stressors and what hormones and neurotransmitters they affect. The stressors can be physical, emotional, and psychological. They can cause what I call the stress response in the body, which is the release of epinephrine, norepinephrine, and cortisol. The stress response affects hormones such as thyroid hormones, estrogen, progesterone, and testosterone. The stressors also have a downstream effect physiologically. When the body responds to stressors by releasing certain hormones and neurotransmitters, it could affect the thyroid gland and cause a slower metabolism, which leads to weight gain.

Scientists are currently working to determine if there could be a correlation between sex hormones and the development of the brain, which later affects how we experience stress. One theory is that our sex hormones' effect on the development of our brain in young adulthood impacts the way we experience stress. What is fascinating about this is that we can retrain our brains to experience the stressors in our lives in a very different way and have them cause a very different reaction on the physiology of our hormones.

Steps to Healing from the Stress

Unless you move to a deserted island or a monastery like I did, you will have stress in your life. It is not necessary to be stressed out as a response to this stress, though. The important thing is to calibrate your stress-o-meter so you can do something about the stress at the very first sign of it. This is the process of becoming empowered to manage your own health care.

The first step is learning exactly where you are right now. Whether or not you experience stress in your life, you may be stressed out. If you are unaware that you are stressed out, you will be less inclined to do something about it. Many women have come to me completely unaware that they were stressed out, just like I was back in medical school. You may have gone to school or worked for years, or you may have stayed at home. There are many types of stressors that your body is always trying to respond to and help keep you in balance with. You need to give yourself and your body a break. Try deviating from the usual pattern and retreat to a place where you are not stressed, or at least not as much as usual, for some time. The key is to relax so that you can come back to your life to see how stressed out you are and identify some tools to better handle your stress.

Relaxing while you are on your journey trying to conceive is essential. It's easier said than done, I know. Realize, though, that even if all of your hormones are completely optimal, you have sex at the exact right time, and you are in the optimal fertile age range, the likelihood of you getting pregnant in any given cycle is 20%. That means only one in five women who have optimal levels of everything is likely to get pregnant in any given month. So there is nothing "wrong" with you just because it doesn't happen the very first time you have unprotected sex. Nothing has to be "wrong" with you even if you have a few months of negative pregnancy tests. When you start on your journey toward family-creation, have patience and give yourself time—a while. It is possible that you will get pregnant the very first time; however, it's rare! Relaxing and releasing the internal pressure you put on yourself, in and of itself, will help support your fertility.

Another important part of understanding your stress is to get your adrenal hormones and neurotransmitters tested by taking a salivary test combined with urinary testing. This type of testing will help you understand where you are right now so that you can find the best way to support your body.

The second step is retraining your body and brain to experience stress differently. For my clients, I use BodyTalk, which I mentioned in an earlier chapter. This modality helps them shift from the sympathetic mode, or the stressed-out state, to the parasympathetic mode, in which the body has the best ability to heal. We do this therapy week after week to retrain their bodies and brains from their usual mode and create a new pattern for responding to stressors in life. In the *Fertility Secrets Bonus Kit*, you will find the video "Cortices," which is a technique for retraining your brain to be in the parasympathetic mode. This technique takes about one minute a day to do, so I highly recommend that you use it to help increase your stress resilience.

The last step is using the appropriate herbs and supplements for your imbalance. This goes back to the first step of understanding where you are and then responding appropriately. Don't take herbs without knowing exactly where you stand. Although the herbs may work great and make you feel more energized, if you take the wrong classification of herbs for your stress response, you may throw your body further out of whack.

Adrenals are the main glands for helping you respond better to stress. There are three stages of adrenal fatigue that you need to understand:

1. The wired stage
2. The wired and tired stage
3. The tired stage.

In Stage 1, there is an excessive response rather than a subdued response. The goal in this stage is to calm down the nervous system that has gone haywire with non-stimulating adrenal herbs. My favorite herbal medicines for this stage are schisandra berries and rose. Both of these combine well with other adrenal support herbs and have a calming, soothing effect on the nervous system, which will go a long way in supporting the adrenal glands. Rose also has a positive effect on the mood, which women with infertility often struggle with.

In Stage 2, the wired and tired stage, you go, go, go, and then crash. Here you want to rebuild and replenish the adrenal energy that has already been depleted while supporting better rest and rejuvenation to nourish the body into a non-tired stage. There is a tricky balance of herbs that help nourish and replenish. My favorite herb here is rhodiola. I usually use it in combination with other herbs—often nutritive herbs such as nettle and fo-ti (a Chinese herb), which help rebuild and replenish the body of nutrients and vitality.

Finally, Stage 3 is the tired stage. This is what most people think of as adrenal fatigue, but it is actually the very last stage, and very few people are at this stage. Here you want to replenish everything that has been depleted. You also want to stimulate the adrenal glands so that they can kick back into gear. So you need herbs that nourish as well as stimulate. In this stage, the traditional adrenal herbs such as eleutherococcus, ginseng, and ashwagandha come in very handy. In this stage too, it is vital to have some nutritive herbs.

It's important to understand these three stages and make sure that the herbs you take to support your body are right for the stage you are in. Testing is important to figure out where you fall and which herbs you should take.

Adrenal health and vitality are at core of optimal fertility. Women who have burnt the candle at both ends for many years are often the ones who struggle with being able to conceive. They often come to me with nutrient deficiencies, weak pulses, and lack of energy or motivation. Some in their earlier stages of fertility challenges are more wired. They try to control the course of action or treatment plan, over-analyze, and are generally overcommitted in their lives— leaving little time for a baby to come in. All these issues, commonly labeled as "stress" or seen as the impact of stress, are factors relating to infertility. Research has shown the impacts of stress on fertility. From my experience, there is more to it than "not stressing." It's almost impossible just to let go of stress sometimes. Building stress resilience is key to helping people live healthier lives and get fertile. The impact that years of stress has had on your body can be healed and reversed with the use of BodyTalk, herbal medicines, and nutrients.

CHAPTER 10

Are You a Mutant?

What We Have Learned from the Human Genome Project

The human genome project—the classification of DNA into a code that we can read, understand, and analyze—has greatly improved our understanding of the genetic makeup of humans, and in turn, it has created many more questions for scientists. Thus far, from the research, we understand that if you have an SNP (or a single nucleotide polymorphism), it simply means that there is one letter that has taken the place of another, changing the outcome altogether. For example, think of the word *cat*. If you change the *U* to an *A*, it *spells cut*, which means something entirely different and may make the whole sentence it appears in incomprehensible! This is exactly what is happening when a letter of a gene sequence is changed. Your body doesn't know or understand how to read it and makes that process either dysfunctional or completely non-functional, depending on how big the error is.

What You Need to Know About MTHFR

Our genetic material has 19,000 to 20,000 protein-coding genes, meaning there are about 20,000 genes that have actual functions in the body. There is, however, a lot of press around one gene in particular: MTHFR (methylenetetrahydrofolate reductase). If you have been struggling with getting pregnant or have had recurring miscarriages, MTHFR has undoubtedly popped up on your radar, so here is what you need to know about it.

MTHFR plays a role in the production of an enzyme that helps the absorption and utilization of folate, which is necessary for the conversion of homocysteine to methionine. This process is also considered important for the methylation pathways in the body.

The gene has variants, or mutants, in two common positions that are tested to determine gene function—the A1298C and C667T. There are more positions that could be tested and analyzed, but these two are pretty informative. These abnormal variants cause a lowered function of these genes. There is a difference between these two variants in reference to fertility, though. The A1298C has lower implications on fertility than the C667T, and if the C667T variant is heterozygous (one mutant), there is about a 30% decrease in gene function, but if they are homozygous (two mutants), there could be up to a 70% drop in functionality.

Although MTHFR is responsible for the conversion of folic acid and folate to 5-MTHF (think of it as active folate), taking folic acid can cause build up and create a backlog in the system if your MTHFR gene is not working correctly. So switch your supplements and prenatal from folic acid over to folate. Also, eat beans, greens, and lentils, which are high in folate and have been shown to be better absorbed and utilized than supplements.

Supplementation is not always the answer, though. If you get this one pathway working well, you could possibly throw off other pathways connected to this one. Besides, if you have an MTHFR variant, you are likely to have other gene SNPs. The key is not just knowing that you have an MTHFR variant but also understanding how all of these pathways work together, where they connect, and which SNPs you have so that you can address all different parts of the function to get your methylation working properly. You can get full genetic profiles through testing via the gene testing and analysis service 23andMe, followed by consulting with a skilled practitioner who understands the various methylation and detoxification pathways and your SNPs in the context of those pathways.

Methylation does the following in the body:

- Supports gene regulation
- Processes hormones
- Processes chemicals and toxins
- Builds immune cells
- Builds neurotransmitters
- Produces energy
- Plays a crucial part in muscle and cell membrane function.

Stress has a big impact on your methylation pathways. It speeds up methylation reactions, so it increases the use of B12, zinc, magnesium, and methionine. High amounts of stress increase the production of epinephrine and norepinephrine, which have to be gotten rid of via methylation. So stress creates a double-whammy on your methylation pathways, and if you don't have enough nutrients or the pathways are blocked, the necessary methylation does not happen. In the cases of high stress, that can keep epinephrine and norepinephrine floating around your body for longer periods of time, impacting different glands and other hormones.

Lastly, 90% of methylation happens in the liver. If your liver is not functioning properly or is "stagnant" as is said in Chinese medicine, it is likely that methylation is not happening as it should. Then things that hinder liver function, such as coffee and alcohol, will decrease proper methylation in the body. As you can see, you can't solve the problem just by supplementing with 5-MTHF.

As if this was not enough, I will add one more layer of complexity to this problem, the complexity of epigenetics. Epigenetics is the expression of gene variation or mutants. You might be a mutant on the inside but not showing any effects on the outside. Why? Because of epigenetics. According to Ben Lynch, "Epigenetic changes are environmentally responsive mechanisms that can modify gene expression independently of the genetic code."[9] Some of the many things that support epigenetic shifts are lifestyle, food, air, exercise, stress, chemicals, xenobiotics (foreign chemical substances found in the body that are not naturally produced in the body such as drugs, hormones, and pollutants), water, heavy metals, and microbiome.

The emergent field of epigenetics offers a lot of hope because it says that just because you have a variant, you don't have to have abnormal function. If the gene expression is hindered by the environment, it can also be supported by the environment. And all the things that I share in this book help support optimal gene expression! So don't make yourself crazy worrying if you're a mutant. There are some cases in which it's important to get genes tested. If you experience repeat miscarriages, unexplained infertility without any other symptoms or hormonal imbalances, or estrogen dominance, I would highly recommend getting your genes tested. Otherwise, relax and trust that the things you're doing to support your health and fertility are also

---

9   Lynch, B. (2014). Maternal and Pediatric Implications due to MTHFR and Methylation Dysfunction [PowerPoint slides]. Retrieved August 2, 2017, from www.seekinghealth.com/media/ICA-MTHFR.pptx

helping support optimal gene function. If you're going to go down the genetic rabbit hole, make sure you're walking hand in hand with someone who has a flashlight and can help support you to get to the other side!

CHAPTER 11

The Secrets Your
Doctor Didn't Tell You

A lot of the fears and frustrations that couples come in with have to do with confusion about their test results and why they're not getting pregnant. They may have some anger because they feel like they haven't been treated well by their doctors, ob-gyns, or reproductive specialists. At that point, they are at a loss of what to do next. They want to partner with their doctors on their fertility journey, and they long to be empowered with knowledge about their bodies and feel hope that they can conceive. A lot of that can be achieved by having a doctor who does the full gamut of blood tests and other tests and gives or points to solutions that address all the issues they have identified.

I recently had a 33-year-old patient who had been struggling to conceive for about a year. She had gone to her ob-gyn, who had run some basic blood tests, and when she had come in to review the results, the ob-gyn had told her that the reason for her difficulty getting pregnant was that she was not ovulating. After the consultation with the ob-gyn, she had begun doing some online research to figure out how the doctor had come to that conclusion. When she came to me, I asked her if her doctor had tested her post-ovulation progesterone levels. She gave me a blank gaze and said she didn't think so. Looking over the blood work, I saw no hormonal testing; all I saw was a very basic blood chemistry panel that didn't have any information on her fertility. When we tested her hormones, it turned out that she was ovulating just fine. So we dug deeper, and we discovered that she had high levels of inflammation and nutrient mal-absorption, which was the likely cause of her infertility.

What Doctors Usually Test

Even though patients think they are getting tested thoroughly, they usually are not. I always ask my patients to bring in lab results from the tests that their previous doctors have done. When I ask them what they have been tested for previously, most aren't sure but say that their doctors told them they have been tested for everything. The truth is that when doctors say they have tested everything, what they may be saying is that they have tested everything the insurance company is willing to pay for and everything they think is reasonable for your signs and symptoms. Most conventional doctors don't believe in testing before you have any symptoms, and although I consider infertility a symptom, other doctors often don't share that opinion and don't want to do more tests and analysis to get to the root of the "problem."

I recently asked my doctor to scan me for a gamut of hormones because I'm getting older and would like to have children at some point. She responded by telling me that I didn't need any of those tests because I didn't have any indications of hormonal irregularities and I hadn't been trying to conceive for at least six months unsuccessfully. From my perspective, the hormone tests were entirely warranted. I think it's a good idea to have a baseline, and I wanted to make sure that I was in good shape so that when I did try to conceive, it wouldn't be very challenging. After much back and forth, the doctor finally agreed but informed me that I would have to pay out of pocket for these tests that may cost $2,000 to $3,000.

When doctors say that they have tested you for everything, realize that everything to them may not include the exact tests that you need. Lab testing is crucial, but it is imperative that you know exactly what to ask your doctor for and that you advocate for yourself.

Beyond the conventional hormone and blood tests, like a complete blood chemistry panel (CBC), there are many alternative tests. I call them "alternative" because only functional medicine doctors will utilize these tests to customize treatments more progressively. The tests I utilize for individualized fertility care are food sensitivity tests, nutritional analysis, genomic testing, and heavy metal or toxins testing. Unfortunately, these tests are most commonly ordered and understood only by integrative doctors—so you will need to seek out an integrative or functional medicine doctor who can be on your fertility team. All these tests give clinicians like me a fuller perspective on what is happening in patients' bodies and allow us to dig deeper into why they are unable to conceive.

The Normal Range

There is a broad range of interpretations for test results, and the doctors are the interpreters. Any lab testing service has its "within normal limits." The doctors look at the results very quickly to see what is out of range. The problem is that it's a large scale, and it doesn't take into consideration what is optimal, but rather what is normal. The normal range is the average of the lab values of a population of people who don't have any known health issues. This normal range is usually quite vast. For more progressive practitioners such as myself, there is a narrower range of what is considered normal limits. The values need to be interpreted within the context the patients' goals for their health and their symptoms.

One of my patients was a 38-year-old woman who had experienced irregular menstrual cycles her entire life. She was not looking to get pregnant but came in for fertility planning because she wanted to have a child in the next two or three years. Upon testing and uncovering her signs and symptoms, I diagnosed her with PCOS, which would have made her fertility challenging if and when she decided to have children. Even though she had been complaining about irregular menstrual cycles, painful periods, and a few other symptoms her entire life, none of her doctors had bothered testing her hormones to figure out what was going on under the surface. Instead, they had given her birth control pill after birth control pill to try to help control her hormones. Her host of hormonal abnormalities led her to decide that she needed to work with me now, rather than take chances on her fertility later. Six months into her hormonal balancing program, she is living symptom-free, has regular menstrual cycles, and has healed her gut inflammation. These are good signs that we are making progress, and in a few more months, I suspect that her hormone tests should be within normal limits. Assuming she keeps her lifestyle changes, she will likely have an easier time conceiving when she decides she is ready to have a baby.

Another one of my patients was a 33-year-old woman with five years of infertility and two miscarriages. She had a TSH of 2.3, which is considered to be within normal range. She also had antibodies to her thyroid, but the antibodies were never tested because the TSH was within normal limits, only by conventional standards. For me, neither her TSH nor her host of other symptoms were normal. In addition to the miscarriages and infertility she had experienced for five years, she had a whole slew of other symptoms including eczema, hair loss, and chronic fatigue. There were also many other symptoms that pointed to her thyroid not functioning as well as it could. Even though the thyroid hormone was technically within the normal range, it was not optimal, and her thyroid was not functioning optimally either. Optimal TSH for fertility is below 2, ideally 1.5. Since it was clear that her TSH needed help, we went ahead and tested all her thyroid hormones. From the hormones we tested, we found that two out of three of her antibody markers were severely elevated. We also discovered that her immune system was out of whack and was attacking her thyroid glands, so of course, her thyroid levels were sub-optimal. To help her conceive, we needed to tame her immune system and then get her thyroid levels down to optimal. Eventually, she did get pregnant and was able to carry that child to term.

In conclusion, I implore you to advocate for proper testing with your doctors or seek out specialists who can support you so that you can better understand your body's true health. Although doctors who follow the Western medicine model delay hormone testing till you are well into six to 12 months of unsuccessful trying, my experience is that discovering that your hormones are normal helps increase your ability to relax and allow your body to do what it is designed to do, and finding imbalances in your hormones allows you to address these. So why wait?

When you receive the results, you more than likely will not get the full picture because doctors often diagnose based on a generic scale. For that reason, I have included the "Cheat Sheet for Understanding Your Results" in the *Fertility Secrets Bonus Kit* as a bonus to this book that you can use to interpret the results. If you haven't already downloaded your copy, please do. It will help you compare what your doctor thinks is normal with what is considered optimal in the world of functional and naturopathic medicine. What is printed in the guide is the optimal level for all the various hormones. You can also get a second opinion by working with a holistic fertility specialist to interpret your results individually.

If you need to get lab tests that your doctor will not order for you, you can order the tests yourself by using the fertility profiles, titled HFC Fertility Panel Follicular & Luteal Phase, that I have created based on what I deem most important (for United States residents only, unfortunately). Here is the link to order your own tests: www.DirectLabs.com/HFC

The results will be sent directly to you, so you will need an integrative doctor to help you analyze them.

CHAPTER 12

Environmental Toxins

The average couple is constantly exposed to environmental toxins. They wake up in the morning surrounded by electromagnetic frequencies. They have cell phones and likely computers around them, not to mention a bed that might have metal springs inside of it, which conduct the electromagnetic frequencies. Then they jump in the shower and lather on soaps, shampoo, and conditioner—all of which are sufficiently labeled with a host of chemicals. The water in the shower is filled with chlorine, fluoride, and heavy metals that they either inhale or absorb through the skin. After they have gotten out of the shower and dried off, they lather up with lotion—likely more chemicals. Then they brush their teeth, which introduces additional toxins, chemicals, and fluorides into the body. The woman will probably go on to her hair and makeup routine, which involves hair care products and hairspray, as well as concealer, foundation, powder, blush, mascara, and eyeliner—all with their own sets of chemicals. Finally, the couple makes it out the door to breathe in chemicals and toxins from the air, and head to where they work. If the buildings where they work are new, there may be off-gassing toxins from the carpet and furniture that the couple inhales. If the buildings are old, they may have mold that adds another layer of exposure. This is the toxic soup that most Americans float in daily. What is your day-to-day exposure to toxins? Before moving forward, fill out the "Fertility

Toxicity Questionnaire" to understand your toxin exposure. You can find this questionnaire in your *Fertility Secrets Bonus Kit*.

A lot of the fears and frustrations of the couples I help relate to the unknown reason fertility is on the decline. In general, male and female fertility has been declining for the last 50 years or so. A meta-analysis of 61 different studies, representing 15,000 men in 23 different countries, reported an average 50% decline in sperm counts from 116 million to 66 million between 1938 and 1990.[10] Although there is some debate among scientists about the acceptance of these reports, several other studies have been conducted since, finding a trend in decreasing numbers of sperm as well as declining quality of sperm.[11]

Though we don't quite know why fertility is declining, one of the underlying reasons we might link to it is the increasing number of chemicals and toxins in the environment. The toxins are in the air as well as in skin care and makeup. There are also an enormous number of estrogen-like compounds in all the plastic things we purchase as well as the water we drink. We know that there are over 300 different toxins in the cord blood of babies.[12] How many more toxins are floating around in a newborn child? We have no idea.

Test Exposure for Answers

If you have unexplained infertility, meaning you have done the appropriate exploring with a functional fertility doctor, and there is

---

[10] Merzenich, H., Zeeb, H., & Blettner, M. (2010). Decreasing sperm quality: a global problem? *BMC Public Health*,10(1). doi:10.1186/1471-2458-10-24

[11] Kumar, N., & Singh, A. (2015). Trends of male factor infertility, an important cause of infertility: A review of literature. *Journal of Human Reproductive Sciences*,8(4), 191. doi:10.4103/0974-1208.170370

[12] Body Burden: The Pollution in Newborns. (2005, July 14). *EWG*. Retrieved July 11, 2017, from http://www.ewg.org/research/body-burden-pollution-newborns

still no concrete explanation, look into testing your environmental toxin exposure. The test costs a few hundred dollars, but it might give you an answer as to why your partner has low sperm counts, low motility (meaning the sperm are challenged in moving up the fallopian tube to the egg), or abnormal morphology (meaning the sperm do not have optimal makeup to penetrate the egg when they reach it), or even why you have high levels of estrogen that might correlate to the toxins floating around in your body. I find the test to be more useful for men than women because there are more toxins known to affect male fertility than female fertility. In the case where there is a motility or morphology issue with the sperm, this might be one of the earlier tests to look into.

Support the Body

There are too many toxins around to get rid of all of them. My first suggestion is to reduce, reduce, reduce. If you can eliminate the major players, it will go a long way in supporting your fertility. Please make sure to refer to the "Map of Fertility Toxins" that affect male and female fertility, along with where they are usually found so that you can begin avoiding exposure to those toxins. If you haven't found this map already, it's in the *Fertility Secrets Bonus Kit*.

This map is just the tip of the iceberg of toxins that we know affect fertility, male or female. Look at this list and see which of these things you can eliminate or reduce, and then begin getting rid of them. You can dive in as deep as you like, but eliminating some of the common and known fertility toxins will also eliminate many of the other less known toxins from your body.

Just as important as reducing the toxin exposure is making sure that you are helping your body to release the toxins on its own. The liver is one of the major detoxification organs. Support it so it can work at its best getting rid of the toxins in your body. To support your liver in ridding the body of toxins, you can make a castor oil pack and put it on your liver and abdomen. In my *DIY Fertility Hacks* e-book in the *Fertility Secrets Bonus Kit*, you will find directions for castor oil packs. There are also a variety of different supplements that will help support your liver. Two of my favorites are NAC (N-acetyl cysteine) and glutathione. If you are ingesting glutathione, it needs to be in a more absorbable form, such as liposomal glutathione. Otherwise, IV glutathione can be used for guaranteed absorption and utilization in the body. Additionally, dandelion root is a traditional herbal medicine that supports liver function and detoxification. New research also shows that dandelion root has promising benefits on fertility as well, so this might be a great addition to your optimal fertility formula. You can talk to your holistic practitioner about what would be right for you.

The other major detoxification organ is your skin. Infrared sauna, exercise, and other things that help open the pores of your skin will help detoxify your body. *Although, being in high amounts of heat for long periods of time may be contraindicated for male fertility.*

It's also helpful to have a stellar gut, meaning optimal digestion for absorption of nutrients and elimination of toxins. Supporting the gut is a little bit trickier because you want to make sure that you don't have what functional doctors call "leaky gut," which is an inflammation of your intestinal tract. Assuming that all is well, you can use things like psyllium husks or flaxseed that will help bind toxins in the intestinal tract and pull them out of your body.

As an additional bonus, the *"Diva's Detox Guide,"* to be found in your *Fertility Secrets Bonus Kit*, is a great resource to get the specifics of makeup, hair care, and skincare products, along with brands to seek out for the purest ingredients. It's not exhaustive by any means, but it's a great place to start and learn what you need to look for on labels.

CHAPTER 13

Let's Not Forget the Men

Although men are the other half of the fertility equation, they are more likely than not just looked at as the sperm donors, the sidebar in the conversation of being able to conceive. I disagree with this perspective. I believe that men are an essential piece of the equation and that looking at them as sperm donors devalues their part in this journey. This journey is equally emotionally rough for the men as the women. Many men have sat in my office expressing their fears, grief, anxieties, and aloneness that they can't express to their wives. As a practitioner, I believe it's important to pay attention and make space for them. Additionally, since IVF has the ability to isolate and select sperm, it bypasses the need for healthy sperm. Sperm is, however, an indicator of male health and vitality, so in a more holistic approach, male health is equally essential to fertility success.

Besides helping with the obvious factors of increasing sperm counts and sperm quality, I have witnessed a few stunning transformations in men. One of my favorites is the one of a 49-year-old man with chronic back pain who came into my office unable to sit or bend down to pick up his 3-year-old child. He and his wife had been unable to conceive since the last child, and the doctors couldn't understand why because all his lab results looked normal. After working with the wife for a while, I started to wonder if I had missed something because besides her minor inflammation that had begun to subside, nothing should have kept her from conceiving. I started shifting my focus over to the man, and I realized that the source of his back pain might be the root cause of their challenge. He was almost 50 years old, and he was very fearful that he would end up an older dad like his father had been, unable to play with the child as he or she grew up. As we peeled away the layers of emotion and fear, his back pain started to lessen, and he regained movement, flexibility, and ability to sit instead of being limited to standing and lying down. After about six weeks of treatment, his back pain subsided, and he regained a full range of motion. Two weeks after that, his wife came to my office thrilled to report that she was pregnant.

You might wonder what this man's back pain had to do with their fertility and how the release of emotions helped them. I don't know if his emotions had been blocking their fertility, but I do know that the couple does not care if they were or weren't—they only care that they now have the second child that they had wanted so much.

Important Tests for Men

There are a couple of tests that are important for men. One is Hemoglobin A1c, which is an estimate of blood sugar levels over three months. Higher-than-normal blood sugar levels over long periods of time usually lead to poor sperm quality. Another test is Kruger Strict sperm analysis. A basic sperm count is okay, but it does not offer much insight into how well the sperm are performing. The Kruger Strict analysis will offer information on the following factors:

- Morphology—the shape, size, and "normality" of the sperm—which points to potential nutritional deficiencies, usually antioxidants

- Motility—the sperm's ability to move quickly through the cervix—which points to potential nutritional deficiencies that may or may not be antioxidant-related

- Agglutination—if the sperm are sticking together—which points to inflammation or high blood sugar levels in men.

If the Kruger Strict analysis results are abnormal, I usually dig further into functional nutritional deficiencies and genetic analysis to get a deeper understanding of what might be underlying the sperm abnormalities.

How to Improve Sperm Health

Now, let's look at some ways to improve sperm health.

First of all, take the SpectraCell micronutrient test. This is a functional medicine test that analyzes and reports the exact levels of nutrients absorbed in the body. This blood test assesses about 30 different minerals, antioxidants, amino acids, and vitamins in the body, and this test can be useful for men and women. Specifically for men, poor antioxidant status is a well-documented cause of male infertility. Free radicals can damage both the sperm's genetic material (which could lead to higher rates of miscarriage) and their cell membranes (which may lead to the sperm being unable to penetrate the egg), and antioxidants can serve as protection from these potential damagers. There are many nutrients that have been researched to improve sperm quality, but I believe that taking all of them might be overkill. It's more important to know the exact nutrients each particular person needs and increase or balance those levels. Nutrients that have been studied to support sperm health are:

- CoQ10, which protects sperm from damage and has been found to increase sperm count and motility

- L-carnitine and acetyl-L-carnitine, which transports fatty acids to the sperm as their preferred energy source and has been shown to increase sperm motility in clinical trials
- Vitamin C, which has been proven to help increase sperm counts, motility, and morphology
- Vitamin E, which has been shown to protect sperm cell membranes, which, in turn, improves the sperm's ability to penetrate the egg
- Selenium, which helps the maturation of sperm and protects sperm from oxidation
- Zinc, which can help increase sperm counts and support testosterone levels.

Second, discover exposure to heavy metals or toxins. If you suspect exposure to heavy metals or any of the toxins listed in the toxins guide you downloaded, the toxins and heavy metals test is essential.

Third, don't cook your balls. This seems obvious, but do not overheat the body. The high temperatures in hot tubs and saunas may affect the testes' ability to do their job. On a similar note, tight underwear is too constricting for optimal blood flow, so take note, men.

CHAPTER 14

Inflammation

In addition to the fear of not getting pregnant, you may fear miscarriage after conception. Once you get a positive pregnancy test, you want to carry the baby to term. Unfortunately, miscarriages, even multiple miscarriages, are relatively common, and there is often no explanation for them.

Inflammation has often been labeled as the secret killer. At this point, most major illnesses from heart disease to cancer to diabetes have been related to a higher-than-normal degree of inflammation in the body. The ability to carry to term is called fecundity, and low fecundity has also been connected to inflammation, often in the gut.

I had a 32-year-old client with a history of three miscarriages in her early trimester. She wanted to conceive naturally, but she was deathly afraid of another miscarriage. Her problem was not getting pregnant but staying pregnant. We discovered that she had several food sensitivities that showed up as eczema. Even though they had been present for a good portion of her life, her other doctors had never connected her fecundity to her gut health. Once we discovered what foods she reacted to, and we removed them from her diet and healed her gut, she was able to get pregnant and carry to term.

Inflammation and Fertility

Research has shown that some of the conditions related to infertility or low fecundity are heavy use of non-steroidal anti-inflammatories such as Aspirin and Tylenol, ulcerative colitis, Crohn's disease, irritable bowel syndrome, leaky gut, and microbiome deficiency. Research also suggests that chronic inflammation brings about pregnancy complications such as gestational diabetes, high blood pressure, and pre-term labor. Women who managed to conceive while diagnosed with inflammatory bowels also showed an increased tendency to deliver pre-term, had a lower birth rate, and delivered more often through C-section. The babies were also small for their gestational age.

Men are not exempt from inflammatory conditions and decreased fertility. In one study, men with inflammatory bowel conditions had a slightly lower fertility rate than a control group. It was noted that these men had a low semen quality—lower sperm motility, sperm concentration, and sperm volume as well as total count. The semen quality decreased by 46% compared to men with no inflammatory bowel condition.

All of this is to say that gut inflammation, mainly chronic inflammation, can cause infertility. Chronic inflammation prevents exertion of essential micro and macronutrients necessary for successful conception and maintaining the pregnancy to term. Low microbial volume and poor dietary choices are also contributing factors to gut inflammation.

Leaky Gut

Leaky gut is a gut inflammation that often brings about inflammation throughout the body. It is usually caused by diseases such as celiac disease and candida and parasite infection. Other causes of leaky gut include prolonged stress, poor diet, alcohol consumption, allergies, some medications (especially non-steroidal anti-inflammatories that I mentioned earlier), steroids, some hormones including oral contraceptives, deficient stomach acid secretions, and an imbalance of the microorganisms in the gut.

Poor nutritional status is both a cause and result of leaky gut. As I said above, poor diet may bring about chronic inflammation, which may impair exertion of the micro and macronutrients that are responsible for facilitating easy conception and successful pregnancy. For example, absorption of protein, fats, zinc, vitamin D, iron, and selenium, which are all important for conception and healthy pregnancy, are largely affected in cases of leaky gut syndrome.

While a normal gut promotes absorption of only digested, beneficial matter into the body, a leaky gut absorbs all matter, including that which has not been digested and may not be usable for the body, as well as toxins that are not meant to be absorbed. The body's immune system reacts to the unwanted materials in the bloodstream. It has a negative effect on near and distant organs and glands, including those of the reproductive system, which may bring about infertility.

Autoimmunity is another adverse effect of a leaky gut. It increases the likelihood of the female body to classify the male sperm as foreign matter, causing an immune reaction to the sperm. This low tolerance to sperm may hinder successful conception. Autoimmunity also increases the chances of hormonal imbalances and may lead to low fecundity. It is often the cause of low implantation rate, and it may also be connected to a higher rate of miscarriage.

Steps to Healing

What can you do about inflammation, leaky gut, and your gut health? First, take tests to check your gut health. Do it before conception. A good test to start with is hs-CRP (high-sensitivity C-reactive protein, which is a marker for generalized inflammation) along with a test to check for antibodies to the thyroid. If either of these is elevated, there is likely some inflammation at the gut level.

Second, get functional tests for assessing your nutritional status. A lab called SpectraCell analyzes nutritional status on the cellular level, beyond what is in your bloodstream. There are also labs that analyze gut permeability and food sensitivities. These might be important in assessing the health of your gut, so working with a functional medicine doctor will be essential to assessing and healing underlying inflammation.

Third, heal the gut microbiome to decrease overall inflammation. It goes beyond taking a probiotic—although that might be a good start. If you are taking a probiotic, make sure it is of good quality. A good quality probiotic has a variety of microorganisms, not just the lactobacillus GG. Look for ones with 10 to 20 varieties of microbes. Also, look for products that have a list of "other ingredients" that is short or non-existent. As a practitioner, I also check how they produced the probiotic. If it was exposed to heat, there are probably no viable organisms. Talk to your holistic fertility doctor about the right products for you. Beyond taking a probiotic, it is beneficial to support the gut microbiome by doing the following:

1. Eat plenty of fiber. Fiber feeds the healthy gut microbes. Some studies suggest that Paleo diets cause a deficiency of fiber that may lead to imbalances.

2. Avoid glyphosates found in an herbicide called RoundUp. It's still being studied, but it is very likely that glyphosates increase the resistance of the not-so-good bacteria and kill off the good stuff,[13,14] causing an imbalance in the precious microbiome.

---

[13] Krüger, M., Shehata, A. A., Schrödl, W., & Rodloff, A. (2013). Glyphosate suppresses the antagonistic effect of Enterococcus spp. on Clostridium botulinum. *Anaerobe*,20, 74-78. doi:10.1016/j.anaerobe.2013.01.005

[14] Samsel, A., & Seneff, S. (2013). Glyphosate's Suppression of Cytochrome P450 Enzymes and Amino Acid Biosynthesis by the Gut Microbiome: Pathways to Modern Diseases. *Entropy*,15(4), 1416-1463. doi:10.3390/e15041416

3. Avoid GMO foods.

4. Reduce your intake of sugar. Sugar feeds only particular bacteria in the gut that can create further imbalances.

5. Eliminate processed foods from your diet. Processed foods don't have the fiber that is available in the wholesome form of those foods.

6. Don't take antibiotics unless necessary. They kill all the bacteria in your body, whether harmful or beneficial, and hence leave your gut vulnerable to microbiome imbalance.

7. Relax while you eat to digest your food better.

These are some of the steps you can take to heal your gut, decrease the inflammation in your body, and help support your fertility as well as fecundity so that you can have a healthy child.

Conclusion

Having a healthy child can be one of our deepest desires, so trying to conceive and not being able to get pregnant can bring up a deep-seeded fear of not being able to have the baby you badly want. It can also bring to the surface some underlying patterns of being uncertain that you're "good enough." As I have noticed with many clients over the years, the disappointment of trying and not being able to conceive gets deeper with every menstrual cycle. And when the infertility is not explained, and the root cause has not been figured out, it can be challenging to keep trying.

Instead of considering infertility as a disease or diagnosis, I look at it as a symptom, so when I treat couples for infertility, I try to figure out the root cause and bring them to a state of health and balance. Over the course of this book, we have explored many of the possible underlying causes of infertility such as hormonal imbalances, inflammation, and poor gut health. There can be many other underlying causes as well.

After I have understood the root cause of infertility, I use a treatment program that follows three foundational principals: detoxify, rebalance, and nourish. Each couple may need to rebalance different things, so every couple needs a unique approach and treatment plan.

In the detoxification phase, we remove things that are influencing the body with toxins that could be causing hormonal imbalances and keeping the body from producing good-quality eggs or sperm. In general, I suggest detoxifying the body every six months. Detoxing is, however, contraindicated during pregnancy and breastfeeding. So it is wonderful to support your body through a detox at least two to three months before conception. There are many different ways to detoxify the body—and I recommend different methods depending on the patient and their body type. It is ideal to work with a practitioner who understands your body and what kind of detox would best support you, rather than using a generic, "detox in a box"-type approach. Also in the detoxification period, we generally support patients to detoxify from the effects of long-term hormonal birth control use. The approach I use for this is the Lalor protocol, which is a series of homeopathic remedies that help remove the energetic impacts of hormone use.

In the rebalancing phase, we rebalance hormones, replete nutrients to their optimal levels, and align the location of the uterus and ovaries for optimal blood flow and health. Last but not least, we rebalance the mind and emotions. Infertility is often an emotional journey with lots of ups and downs, and it can bring up insecurities or patterns from childhood. This is the perfect time to heal those underlying patterns so that they don't carry on to your future children.

After the mind, body, and spirit are rebalanced, it is important to nurture and nourish the body with positive thoughts, good food, and essential nutrients that are necessary for the development of the baby. This will support you throughout the cycle until conception and continue supporting a balanced well-being throughout pregnancy.

I have shared various tips and advice to help your fertility. If you get nothing else from this book, I hope you will at the very least use the following three tips that are vital to your fertility: First, understand your body and cycle by tracking your basal body temperatures. Measure your temperature as soon as you wake up every morning to gather information. Second, get your hormones tested early on so you can have peace of mind and allow your body to do what it is designed to do or address any imbalances. Finally, relax and be patient with yourself because that in itself will help support your fertility.

If you are actively trying to have a baby but have "unexplained infertility" or want to get to the root of why you are not able to get pregnant or stay pregnant, I suggest filling out the quiz "How Fertile Are You?" This quiz is a great starting point for discovering the potential underlying issues that have made it challenging for you to get pregnant or carry to term. Next, invest in yourself and your future child. Get the support you, and your partner, need to create a healthy body, mind, and spirit. Finally, continue nourishing your body throughout conception and pregnancy.

Most people who have been told that they or their eggs are too old or that IVF is their only option are just not fully supported in understanding and healing their bodies. I believe that if you have a regular, healthy menstrual cycle, and you don't have any structural abnormalities that would keep you from conceiving and carrying to term, you likely can have a healthy baby.

Even IVF is usually more successful if the body is in an optimal state of balance before going into the IVF cycle, so if you choose IVF, it's wise to take the time to rebalance your body first. It saves you pain, heartache, time, and money in the long run. I have worked with couples that have had multiple failed IVF or IUI cycles. I truly believe that the reason they are more successful with my approach is that we are getting to the underlying problem and treating and rebalancing those imbalances rather than trying to control the hormones to make conception happen. This approach generally leaves couples in a healthier, happier state and leads to a natural progression to conception and carrying to term.

As you have read this book, I hope you have learned more ways to support your fertility and carry to term. Follow the recommendations, download the additional resources, and help yourself shift your lifestyle to a more fertile one. If you're looking to conceive sooner rather than later, find the best person or team to support your mind, body, and spirit to morph into a fertile state. I believe that is possible for you.

On your journey, you can impact both future and past generations. You have the opportunity to affect not only your own child's health but also the health of your grandchildren. Use the healing of your womb to reach an optimal state of health to positively impact the health of your child and the health of the genes and seeds of a future child within its embryo. The fertility journey may also call for healing of imbalances in your ancestors. Even if your ancestors are no longer in their bodies, they can receive healing through your healing, so with your journey, you may affect them. Hence, the Native American perspective that healing yourself is healing seven generations through you is true. Open up to the opportunity to heal and transform, and surrender to the possibility of optimal health and living your fullest potential.

May you find success in creating the life and family you envision for yourself.

About the Author

Aumatma Shah was born in India, and at the age of 9, she and her family moved to New Jersey, where she grew up. She went on to obtain an undergraduate degree in biology at Rutgers University while being equally called to studying religion and psychology and attempting to integrate those three fields.

After her undergraduate degree, she discovered her calling in naturopathic medicine, which is founded on the integration of body, mind, and spirit. She pursued a dual degree in naturopathic medicine and a master's in nutrition at the University of Bridgeport, Connecticut. She mentored with many prominent doctors on the East Coast and in India in addition to obtaining her degrees.

For the last 10 years, she has lived and practiced in Northern California, serving the world in a way that her spirit calls her to serve. In 2015, she was named the Bay Area's "Best Alternative Medicine Practitioner." These days, in addition to transforming the lives of the couples that work with her, she is working long distance with clients in a group setting to help them conceive. She is also developing a technology that is bound to change the future of women's health, women's relationships with their bodies, and the awareness of women's hormones and hormonal balance.

You can connect with Dr. Aumatma on her website: www.draumatma.com. Join her email list so that you can stay in touch. For direct communications, you can email her at doc@holisticfertilitycenter.com.

Made in the USA
Middletown, DE
09 May 2023